Teen Success!

Ideas to Move Your Mind

2nd Edition

Beatrice J. Elyé

Great Potential Press™

Teen Success!: Ideas to Move Your Mind, **2nd Edition**

Cover Design: M W Velgos Design
Interior Design: The Printed Page
Edited by: Jennifer Ault

Published by
Great Potential Press, Inc.
P.O. Box 5057
Scottsdale, AZ 85261
www.giftedbooks.com

© 2007 by Great Potential Press, Inc.
Printed and Bound in the United States of America

10 09 08 07   5 4 3 2 1

Library of Congress Cataloging-in-Publication Data

Elyé, Beatrice J. (Beatrice Josephine), 1928-
  Teen success! : ideas to move your mind. — 2nd ed. / Beatrice J. Elye.
     p. cm.
  Rev. ed. of: Jumpstart : ideas to move your mind / Beatrice J. Elyé with Catherine A. Southwick.
  Includes bibliographical references and index.
  ISBN-13: 978-0-910707-83-1
  ISBN-10: 0-910707-83-9
  1. Teenagers—Life skills guides. I. Elyé, Beatrice J. (Beatrice Josephine),
1928- Jumpstart. II. Title.
  HQ796.E567 2007
  646.700835—dc22
                              2007036814

ISBN-13: 978-0-910707-83-1
ISBN-10: 0-910707-83-9

Dedication

This book is dedicated to my first and best teachers—my parents,
to all the students I had the privilege of teaching,
to my encouraging friends,
and to many wonderful librarians.

Acknowledgments

Writing *Teen Success* would have been an insurmountable challenge without the help of Catherine Ann Southwick. In our many discussions concerning its content, we established wonderful rapport and often spent hours evaluating the appropriateness of a single word. Both of us hunted for quotations that would amplify and extend the meaning of the ideas in each chapter. She provided a contemporary viewpoint that made the selection process of these quotations a challenge. I hereby acknowledge her capable determination, valuable insights, and intellectual integrity; without her help, this book might never have been published.

Another friend and esteemed colleague, Carol Hibbard, critically reviewed each of the original chapters. With her wisdom and language skills, she spent many hours perusing both the original papers upon which this book is based and some of the final rewritten chapters. Her careful and intelligent critique resulted in changes that have made the reading easier and more informative.

I am grateful to Dr. James T. Webb and the editors at Great Potential Press, Inc. for their invaluable help in preparing this book for publication.

Finally, I owe major gratitude to a large number of those creative people who informed my life with their wit and insight. Their creative expressions expanded my knowledge of the human condition. They have given me alternative ideas and showed me by their choices that living is a selective process where decisions may be influenced by cultural and societal experiences. I especially admire people who fulfill their promise despite handicaps or difficult circumstances. One of my heroes is Nelson Mandela; therefore, it seems appropriate to quote a selection from his 1994 inaugural speech. These powerful words describe his sense of what thoughtful people must do. His words also suggest how and why I will be thankful if this book has meaning for you.

Our deepest fear is not that we are inadequate. Our deepest fear is that we are powerful beyond measure. It is our light, not our darkness that most frightens us.

We ask ourselves, "Who am I to be brilliant, gorgeous, talented, and fabulous?" Actually, who are you not to be? Your playing small does not serve the world. There's nothing enlightened about shrinking so that other people won't feel insecure around you.

As we let our own light shine, we unconsciously give other people permission to do the same.

– Nelson Mandela

Contents

Preface

This book is based on material that I used as a teacher of high school students, ages 14 to 18, who were doing well in school—either achieving high grades or obviously possessing special talents. These students were full of idealism and dreams for the world and their future, but they often lacked experience and skills in areas like time management and decision making that would make them effective leaders. I realized that a book of ideas based on my experiences could help high school and college students, as well as many adults, to improve their mental, creative, and self-management skills.

I had dreams for every student I taught. I wanted each of them to be happy, to enjoy learning enough to ache for it, to live an examined life, and to make decisions based upon personal ethics. I hoped they would prize honesty. I wanted my students to be blessed with good friends and to treasure family. In retrospect, I realize that I did not care if they became "successes" in the competitive modern sense of that term, but I always expected them to do their best at whatever they did.

For their sake, and that of future generations, I wanted my students to appreciate both the beauty of the earth and its fragility, especially as an environment for all forms of life. I tried to share with them what I treasure—the ability to reason and the desire to delight in the amazing insights provided by scientists, writers, artists, and musicians, among others. I wanted them to learn that every experiment is a personal trip into the unknown, with guidelines of observation and analysis of data as their only compass. Furthermore, I wanted them to understand that experimentation is the fundamental basis of each person's life journey; every day contains new adventures and experiments that shape us.

I believe that everyone has talent. I also believe that all of us must use whatever mental abilities we possess wisely and without arrogance. Just as we benefit daily from the efforts of all of those who have preceded us—using their discoveries and enjoying their creative works—so are we obliged to provide future generations with the fruits of our creative efforts.

Using and developing one's abilities should not simply be drudgery, however. To me, there is a joy within the search process that accompanies creative effort—a pleasure that I tried to impart to my students, and a joy that I now hope to share with those who read this book.

How to Use This Book

Although many books assume that one chapter builds on preceding ones, this book does not. You do not need to read the chapters in sequence. Instead, you can choose chapters based on your personal needs or a chapter's appeal. Exceptions are the first chapter, titled "Personal Notebooks," which is referred to throughout the book, and the last chapter, "All of Your Tomorrows," which contains references to previous chapters. You may want to scan the Table of Contents, as well as the summary at the end of each chapter, in order to locate material that appeals to you.

I have selected topics based on their importance to a creative life. Some of the chapters may help you with practical activities, such as speed reading. Other chapters provide useful information on managing personal problems, such as frustration. Still other chapters discuss thought processes, such as decision making.

I suggest reading each chapter at a pace that allows you to complete the recommended exercises or activities before proceeding to the next chapter. Because each chapter could "stir the mind" initially for as much as one to two weeks, include time to complete, reflect, and assimilate.

Because a broad base of information is important, I have highlighted ideas, people, and events about which you may wish to gather more information by inserting the symbol: 📖. In addition, I have purposely used some words that are nowadays common among well-educated people. You may wish to look them up to better understand their meaning and context. Because these words are often used by knowledgeable people, don't just skip over the ones you do not know.

The following suggestions may help you get the most out of *Teen Success*:

1. Quickly scan the chapter to locate citations containing the 📖 symbol, and gather materials or references you will need to research them. You may enjoy doing an Internet search. Doing research outside of your normal range of interests will help you

extend your knowledge. Also, locate a good dictionary in which to look up new words you read.

2. Reread the chapter more slowly this time. Use the reference materials you have collected to assist in understanding the concepts. Develop any ideas suggested by the chapter.

3. Attend events at local cultural institutions as suitable sources of inspiration and/or rewards for your hard work.

In this book, I have included much wisdom imparted from others. You may not be familiar with many of the people who are quoted. Each of these people led fascinating lives, and you might enjoy doing some research about them. Three aids in each chapter will help you search for information, both now and in the future:

▣ The brief summary near the end of each chapter allows you to locate general content.

▣ The "Index of Names" at the end of the book lists the names of people mentioned in the text, including authors of cited books.

▣ The "Index of Quotations" lists authors and the first words of their quotes as they appear throughout this book.

Your Journey

You may have wonderful dreams that can be realized by using some of the suggestions in this book. I hope that *Teen Success* will be a book that you will write in, and that you will personalize it and expand it with your own ideas as you read the various chapters. At some future time, you may enjoy rereading sections, especially because your comments may trigger new thoughts and changes in your life's direction. Your notes may give you a sense of who you were, who you are now, and how you have grown. Upon rereading, you may say to yourself, "Did I really write this or think that?" And on the journey of life—that adventure with so few signposts—perhaps you will come to better know yourself.

Finally, you are entitled to know something about my philosophy and beliefs. The core of what I consider important, relative to this book, is the following:

- Life is a journey of self-discovery, a learning experience. Honesty is the mirror I must use to search my innermost being. A quote from Shakespeare's *Hamlet* says it well: "This above all. To thine own self be true, and it must follow, as the night the day, thou canst not then be false to any man."

- My life depends on how I manage it daily—moment by moment. No one else should be held accountable more than I for any part of my life (assuming that I am able to think and am in reasonable health). I am not suggesting that I have complete freedom; no one does. But I can respond sensibly to challenges, problems, and opportunities, even when I do not have control of a situation. I may need to be inventive, and there will be occasions when I am overwhelmed; then I must accept help.

- I am not able to change until I am ready to be influenced. In almost all human interaction, the readiness factor is the basis of meaningful change. For example, learning is a shared responsibility, a contract between student and teacher.

- Life should be joyous and have many moments of happiness. Bubbles of laughter are yeast for my creativity—a satisfying part of my life. I must actively pursue happiness.

- I must treasure life. This means being thoughtful in all human interactions, being kind to all life, and respecting that which supports life—the environment. When I fail, as I will on occasion, I must seek to correct my mistakes.

The items in my list are not ranked in any particular order—all are equally important; any one may predominate in a particular situation. Perhaps your own set of beliefs will become clearer to you as you read this book.

This book is a collection of insights culled from my own experiments in living. I enjoy being creative, and I have developed various skills both by joining scholarly pursuits and by seeking innovative activities. Some of the events in my life could have been overwhelming if I had used less thoughtful methods of reacting to problems. Instead, I not only found ways to take pleasure in what was possible, but I also often managed to convert the possible into improbable good fortune. My life has been a marvelous adventure. I hope you will find some of my ideas useful to your adventuring. I wish you the best of journeys.

Chapter 1

Personal Notebooks: A Key Resource

Throughout history, many famous and creative people have kept notebooks to record their reflections and experiences, among them Leonardo da Vinci 📖 and Charles Darwin 📖. You don't need to be famous, however, to find keeping a notebook helpful. I believe you will find it invaluable in improving your observational and creative thinking skills and in understanding and planning your life.

Your choice for a notebook depends upon your plan for using it. Small, pocket size notebooks are ideal for being constant companions. Larger ones provide more space for writing and can be kept in some convenient special place such as a bedside table, desk, or locker. Ruled paper, art sketchbooks, or bound blank paper books all have various advantages and are commercially available. Computers may be used as well.

The most important part of your notebook is not its form but rather its content. Your purpose in journaling should be to record ideas. That is, this journal is not the diary-type to record what you did when or where, nor is it the classroom information-type, useful for fact retrieval. Instead, it is primarily for your personal observations, thoughts, and concepts.

Try the following. Think of something that interests you—something that you wish to make or do, a problem, or something that you hope to understand. Write it in your notebook. Then, think about it in your spare moments, persistently. Consider or fantasize all kinds of possibilities or solutions, and write them in your notebook. Wherever you are, look at different objects and try to find how they might relate to your idea or problem. Your ideas may seem wild, silly, or even apparently hopeless, but record them anyway. Let your mind freely explore, and describe your thoughts in your notebook.

This process of describing, which allows you to focus on your creative idea, could be verbal, pictorial, or musical. Let your descriptions be both expansive and passionate. *The Grand Canyon Suite* 📖, *Mood Indigo* 📖, and *Ebbtide* 📖 are each musical descriptions. Picasso's *Guernica* 📖 is a powerful pictorial description of his reaction to the bombing of the Basque capital in the Spanish Civil War. It is a masterpiece depicting the agony of war.

Ideas recorded in your notebook—however sketchy, brief, or tentative—can be the initial stage of eventually finding something worth transforming into concrete form. Of course, you may not use any of your early ideas, but the practice of writing and describing your concepts is a useful exercise to make your future efforts at creativity easier and more valuable to you and others. Remember, at this point, you need not be concerned with the practicality of your entries. Techniques for evaluating ideas are suggested in other chapters of this book.

You can use your notebook for a variety of purposes. Include in it any appealing tidbit that can be creatively rearranged or thought about in a new context. You may wish to note ideas or actions that seem innovative and useful. For example, you might imagine how some household items could be recycled into usable objects or how you might reorganize some part of your daily life. Perhaps you might describe or diagram these topics in your notebook.

You could set aside a part of your notebook to record unusual information that appeals to you, such as famous quotations, news events, bits of conversation, descriptions, or unusual words or terms. Many authors maintain records of chance conversations overheard in public places because they like the phrasing or wish to make sure they remember the concepts.

You might also set aside a portion of your notebook for poetry and other metaphorical writing. Writing poetry is a great mind-sharpener. Anton Chekhov's 📖 advice to his brother is worthwhile: "In descriptions one must seize upon small details, grouping them so that when the reader closes his eyes, he gets a picture. For instance, you'll have a moonlit night if you write that on the mill dam a piece of glass from a broken bottle glittered like a bright star." You could write a daily aphorism such as, "Ships are safe in a harbor; but that is not what ships are made for." Aim at making your notebook personal, imaginative, and perhaps quotable.

Other notebook entries could include a description of something, perhaps written from an imagined viewpoint other than your own. How would a worm describe daily events seen along the edge of a pond? This requires "double think"—not just what you would sense, but what someone or something else would sense.

Whether or not you are artistic, attempt to sketch something from your surroundings. Do this on a regular basis to sharpen your observation skills.

From the newspaper or Internet, select and focus on an issue that interests you. Social, political, scientific, and artistic problems abound. Imagine that you are in a position to work on that problem. Use your notebook to brainstorm your ideas and to summarize whatever relevant information is available. Record your opinions regarding this problem. Talk to a variety of people about these issues. Perhaps you may wish to write letters to people who are in a position to influence the problem, and include these letters in your notebook.

Remember to date each notebook entry to provide both a sense of history and perspective. If you think you have an exceptionally good idea, have your record notarized. (Many banks have personnel who can notarize material for little or no cost.) This would be valuable in case you later wish to make a patent or copyright application. For this reason, make sure that your notebook is bound in such a way that pages cannot be inserted or removed unless binding or paging is affected.

Above all, remember that your personal notebooks are very special. They are meant to be a source of fun and excitement, not a chore. Ten years from now, they will likely still delight you and may even serve as a source of additional ideas.

Summary

◙ Keep a personal notebook.

◙ Use it to record any ideas that interest you.

◙ Include in your notebook creative responses to ideas.

◙ Reexamine its content occasionally.

Words of Wisdom

I do not think that I will ever reach a stage when I will say, "That is what I believe. Finished." What I believe is alive…and open to growth.…
— Madeleine L'Engle

I think that one's art is a growth inside one. I do not think one can explain growth. It is silent and subtle. One does not keep digging up a plant to see how it grows.
— Emily Carr

Bring ideas in and entertain them royally, for one of them may be the king.
— Mark Van Doren

Man's mind stretched to a new idea never goes back to its original dimensions.
— Oliver Wendell Holmes

Ideas should be received like guests—in a friendly way, but with the reservation that they are not to tyrannize their host.
— Alberto Moravia

Use what language you will, you can never say anything but what you are.
— Ralph Waldo Emerson

The great art of writing is the art of making people real to themselves with words.
— Logan Pearsall Smith

The events in our lives happen in a sequence in time, but in their significance to ourselves, they find their own order… the continuous thread of revelation.
— Eudora Welty

The act of putting pen to paper encourages pause for thought; this in turn makes us think more deeply about life, which helps us regain our equilibrium.
— Norbet Platt

It is necessary to write, if the days are not to slip emptily by. How else, indeed, to clap the net over the butterfly of the moment? For the moment passes, it is forgotten; the mood is gone; life itself is gone. That is where the writer scores over his fellows: he catches the changes of his mind on the hop.
— Vita Sackville-West

Chapter 2

The Time of Your Life: How to Spend Your Time Wisely

Think of all your daily activities, routine and otherwise. What did you do yesterday that makes today a better day? What will you do today? What should you do tomorrow? How are you spending your time?

People often forget that they have a choice; they can manage their time, or they can let other people and events control their time. Consult your priorities. Critically examine your desires, beliefs, and values. What choices have you been making? Do you want to change those choices? Do some hard thinking. It is *your* life.

You can design and implement a pattern to your life—a sense of what you will do and what you won't do. How much time, for example, will you allot for daily work, self-growth, human interaction, health maintenance, or charitable actions?

The previous questions are not easy to answer. But without these answers, your life may be a haphazard journey. No one else can better contribute to making your everyday life not just okay but spectacular. There are only so many spring times, friendships, and bursts of insight in anyone's lifetime. Determine the best way for you to develop a sensibly balanced use of time.

Laying It All Out

Very busy people seem to accomplish more than others do. In fact, a common expression is, "If you want something done, ask a busy person." Why? Because busy people are often more efficient users of their time and can be counted on to get the job done. Everyone has 24 hours in a day, but nearly all of us can learn to use this limited resource more efficiently. The time we waste because we have not planned its best uses is the most costly expenditure of our lives.

This is not to say that time spent idly or doing activities simply for fun is necessarily wasted time—quite the contrary. We all need time to have fun and enjoy ourselves, as well as for rest and reflection. In fact, this is some of the most valuable time we can spend.

However, doing things inefficiently or participating in activities that don't take us in the direction that we'd like our lives to go is time wasted. For instance, handwriting a paper and then typing it on the computer is a two-step process that can be cut to one step if you are the kind of person who can type out your thoughts as easily as you can write them on notebook paper. Or time could be wasted hanging out at the mall with a crowd of peers whose values you disagree with. If their goal is to see who can shoplift without getting caught, then your time is being squandered! As Benjamin Franklin said, "Lost time is never found again."

The first step toward better managing your time is to discover how you currently use it. To do this, make a list of your daily and weekly activities. Most people have an average of about four hours of "discretionary" time (D-Time) per day, sometimes called leisure time. This is time not required for work, school, family-related obligations, or health maintenance, such as exercise or personal hygiene. In your notebook, prepare a chart of the D-Time that you anticipate you will have for a period of at least a week. Now examine the data. Are you satisfied with your time usage? Do you have time to do the things that you find interesting and enjoyable? Are you spending your time doing things that will help you achieve what you want for your future? If not, what would you like to change?

Consider what you really wish to accomplish—this week, this month, this year. Carefully think about your future, your innermost desires, and your talents and abilities. List in your personal notebook three accomplishments that you would like to achieve this year. Don't list more than three; otherwise you will have difficulty seeing what is really important to you. What motivates you? How do you want to live?

Now look back again at your D-Time chart. Is the time management in your present D-Time chart likely to help you achieve those goals? If not, what changes could you effect? Here are some suggestions:

1. Obtain a calendar, or use one on your computer, that has space for you to write daily entries. Within D-Time periods, make

notations or appointments for activities that you think might help you reach your goals. For example, set aside Monday from 4 to 6 p.m. to research colleges known to be strong in the subjects that most interest you. Consider this appointment with yourself to be as important as a doctor's appointment, and don't break it. Regular use of such a calendar to record daily activities is one of the best ways to organize your time.

2. Make lists of ideas related to your goals. Break a larger goal down into smaller goals. If you have your heart set on going to a particular college, write down what you will need to accomplish to get accepted there. What classes will you need to have taken in school? What extracurricular activities or volunteer work will help you gain acceptance? Will you apply for scholarships? Which ones are available directly from the university you have chosen? What colleges will you apply to as backups?

3. If your D-Time for desired activities is hampered by other obligations, be creative. Get up earlier, swap chores with a sibling, or seek ways to save time spent on routine activities. Aim at having better control of all of your time. You may discover that some of your activities are unnecessary but have become habitual. For example, do you eat breakfast in front of the television? Do you wait to leave the house until a particular morning show is over? What could you better do with that time?

4. Schedule recreation and rewards. For instance, if you have satisfactorily completed an essay that was part of your college entrance package, reward yourself by forgetting about colleges for the next weekend and go to the pool with friends instead!

5. Get enough rest. Rest is an important aspect of time management that will help you be happier and more productive.

Don't Forget to Make Time for the Essentials

On the occasion of her hundredth birthday, a woman responded to a reporter's question, "What regrets do you have?" by quickly saying she wished that she had gone dancing and ridden the Ferris Wheel more often.

You may think that this is a strange answer. But what if she had said, "I wish I had washed more dishes." Wouldn't that answer be stranger?

A balanced approach to life includes time for self-growth, work, human interaction, and charitable actions—and, of course, having fun. You should find time to take pleasure in many activities, including those that may seem frivolous. Remember that dancing is good exercise and that Ferris Wheels offer the opportunity of an interesting view and the time to talk to a friend. Furthermore, sharing such recreational occasions with friends and family create memories that may give you strength during troubled times. All work and no play can diminish the quality of your achievements because of a narrowed vision of life or a limit to self-growth and happiness.

Finally, don't forget to schedule time for charitable actions. Giving enriches both the giver and the receiver. Perhaps without you even being aware, we all benefit from the giving of a multitude of people. Those who have contributed to many publicly shared facilities such as schools, hospitals, libraries, art galleries, and radio and television stations have helped everyone—either directly or indirectly. Become personally involved in community enterprises by donating time (as well as money) to help in maintaining civilization.

Summary

- Allocate time thoughtfully.

- Prepare a personal time chart, including D-Time.

- Study your time usage for possible improvement.

- List a few desired accomplishments for this year, and set aside time to work on them.

- Make and use an appointment-type calendar to schedule your time.

- Be sure to schedule rewards.

- Set aside time for both pleasure and charitable actions.

Words of Wisdom

What I do today is important because I am exchanging a day of my life for it.
> – Hugh Mulligan

It's not what you were, it's what you are today.
> – David Marion

The opportunity of life is very precious and it moves very quickly.
> – Ilyani Ywahoo

There is no such thing in anyone's life as an unimportant day.
> – Alexander Woollcott

Ultimately, time is all you have and the idea isn't to save it but to savor it.
> – Ellen Goodman

Time is the coin of your life. It is the only coin you have, and only you can determine how it will be spent. Be careful lest you let other people spend it for you.
> – Carl Sandburg

Time flies over us, but leaves its shadow behind.
> – Nathaniel Hawthorne

Those who make the worst use of their time most complain of its shortness.
> – La Bruyere

When one has much to put in them, a day has a hundred pockets.
> – Fredrick Nietzsche

Each day, and the living of it, has to be a conscious creation in which discipline and order are relieved with some play and pure foolishness.

– May Sarton

They say that time changes things, but you actually have to change them yourself.

– Andy Warhol

Time is a companion that goes with us on a journey. It reminds us to cherish each moment, because it will never come again. What we leave behind is not as important as how we have lived.

– Captain Jean-Luc Picard

Time and tide wait for no man. A pompous and self-satisfied proverb, and was true for a billion years; but in our day of electric wires and water-ballast we turn it around: Man waits not for time nor tide.

– Mark Twain

Half our life is spent trying to find something to do with the time we have rushed through life trying to save.

– Will Rogers

Chapter 3

Observation: What Do You Really See?

How do you know what you know? Are you really aware of yourself and of what is going on around you? Is there a common source for all knowledge? The following scenarios may help you develop answers to these questions. Think about how each scenario differs from the others and what they have in common.

Scenario 1

Unexpectedly, your team has just won a championship. Sweat is pouring down your face. The roar from the crowd chips away your teammates' words as you joyously high five and hug one another. You look toward the bleachers and see faces with incredible clarity. Every part of you is achingly alive.

Scenario 2

Everyone has been blindfolded in an experiment on sensitivity and asked to find a specific chair. Your first task is to determine your position in the room. Physical chaos occurs as people bump into furniture and each other. But by standing still and listening, you hope to find your way to your own chair without colliding with others. It is not an easy activity.

Scenario 3

You gaze into a deep valley overhung with grey clouds spitting tongues of gold. Surrounding you are fields of asters, a scent of sweetness, and the low grumbling sounds of thunder. You snatch a single flower stalk and sweep it around your head with whoops of joy. Then you quickly gather your belongings, including the best water color painting you have ever made, and run for cover before the rain starts.

What did all of these descriptions have in common? Each scene described sensory responses to the environment. Major events, because they are dangerous, exciting, and/or totally engrossing, can increase your sensitivity to your surroundings (Scenario 1). Your observational skills are subconscious and sometimes not acknowledged until they are threatened or changed (Scenario 2). When your senses are stimulated by interesting, beautiful, or unique circumstances, your observations and responses can be extraordinary (Scenario 3).

As a baby, you probably observed that crying brought you attention, and you learned to time your efforts accordingly. When you wanted someone to pick you up, you were willing to expend the energy to cry. Successes reinforced these efforts, and part of your personality may have been forged by those early wails. You learned to observe cause and effect, and these early experiences contributed both to your inventory of observations and to your skill in observing.

Do you remember a time in childhood when a dandelion blossom was worth lengthy, intense observation? That "play" was self-education—your personal discovery of the world. However, formal schooling interfered, to some extent, with your direct sensory experience. In school, opinions, descriptions, and values of others were introduced to you and became substitutes for your own observations of things. Perhaps the sensory pleasures of puffing at dandelion seed heads disappeared—especially when you were told that dandelions are weeds and are undesirable in manicured lawns.

Your ability to observe and explore with a child's eye has diminished. You seldom have the time for direct observation of the real thing. You make do with substitutes such as books, pictures, or models, but these are all secondary sources of information. A book about flowers is not as direct as the flower itself in your hand. A picture of a mountain is not the same as standing before it with your eyes lifted to the summit.

Of course, second-hand information can be beneficial when the real thing is not available. It creates myriad sensory data that are compressed into something—not the real thing, but better than nothing. However, a photograph, even with its problems of scale and incomplete sensory information, can become more real than the object or event represented. A television sequence becomes a "slice of life." When you continuously work with second-hand information, your chances of really seeing—and really knowing—lessen. Vicarious sensing is a crutch that allows you to make do. Superficially, you seem to know more, but the essence of reality is lost.

It is worthwhile to maintain your child's eye perspective, which has few preconceived expectations or biases and which is one of the most important sources of creativity. When events become commonplace, we take them for granted, and often our appreciation of their value diminishes. We recognize objects that we handle daily but without consciously recalling their detail. When you see something, what do you really see? How accurately? With what purpose? With what influence of previous experience? How much are you affected by your cultural background, biological inheritance, and education in any particular observational situation?

Participating in an event such as mountain climbing produces information that is multi-dimensional; you involve all of your senses. Your observations of such a direct experience are vividly emblazoned within your mind. You can build on this knowledge and memory with confidence. You have faith in its validity; you were there. You have obtained "active-sensory" or primary-source knowledge. Such personal experience of the world is preferable, but since it is difficult and time-consuming to directly acquire such sensory knowledge, using secondary sources often is an easier and more practical—though less satisfactory—way to expand what you know.

Watching documentaries or reading about mountain climbing also produces information—of the "passive-sensory" or secondary-source type, but this may not be as accurate. Before you can accept secondary-source knowledge in any new context, you need to be assured that it was obtained by capable people who observed reality directly themselves. Perhaps you have experienced an occasion when someone inaccurately observed one of your actions and thereby caused problems. Such misrepresentations frequently occur between people.

On a worldwide basis, observational errors exist in many areas of interpersonal relations—entrepreneurial, social, political, and diplomatic. Unintentional errors also occur in accepted knowledge sources such as books, newspapers, and the Internet. Erroneous and careless use of secondary-source material is perhaps the greatest modern threat to intelligent living. We live in an era of information overload that makes information summaries appear enticing. This means that in situations where you must use summaries by others (i.e., secondary sources) you need to be vigilant, neither accepting nor rejecting ideas without careful thought.

Consider the following common statements:

1. "I need to see it for myself."

2. "If I am to be a leader, I need to talk directly to the people I will be leading."

3. "I see a play only after I read the reaction of the critics."

4. "I know what the experts say—but if they disagree, how can they be experts?"

5. "She is a teacher, so what she says must be right."

6. "It was on the Internet or in the newspaper, so it must be true."

Examples 1 and 2 refer to active sensory situations. Examples 3 and 4 suggests a skeptical examination of secondary sources. Examples 5 and 6 indicate a possible non-critical acceptance of a secondary source. As a thoughtful person, you will evaluate secondary source summaries for yourself.

Underlying all of your activities and everyday choices is the process of observation. But how you critically examine any observational process will determine whether your observation results in creative insights. Observation—whether from primary or secondary sources—influences your decisions and beliefs and thus indirectly determines what you can accomplish. Consider the politician who maintains direct contact with the people who elect him. He gathers evidence of their needs from conversations with his constituents. Because of his frequent and direct observations, he is more likely to sponsor practical legislation than another politician who has less direct contact with the people who elected him.

Observation serves many purposes, including the ability to identify, locate, and know. How do you know that a particular object belongs to you? What identifying clues do you use? If you had to claim a lost object, how accurately could you describe it?

Ordinarily, such precision in awareness is unnecessary. For example, as you sit reading this, you are probably unaware of the weight of your shoes or clothes or wristwatch—at least you were, until now when your observation is focused on them. Much of what you sense throughout the day becomes static, squelched by a properly functioning biological system. Without such selective awareness, observational overload would occur, and you would become fatigued by the vast number of sensory signals.

You tend to use your senses at varying levels of intensity, much like settings on a stove. The lowest setting is the subconscious. A warmer setting would be the equivalent of normal consciousness. The more that sensory impressions filter into the consciousness, the hotter the setting, until a "red hot" alert takes place and extreme sensitivity occurs. This is why looking at something intensely can lead to an uncommon and particularly keen awareness. However, it is difficult to maintain such intense focus for a long time. Your mind may wander off target. Exercises in concentrated attention and "centering," which have been an important part of Eastern culture for centuries, can help maintain focus. Some of these techniques have entered Western civilization via Zen 📖 publications and centers.

If you wish to explore Zen and its related areas, the following resources can be helpful. One that is particularly interesting is *Zen and the Art of Happiness*, by Chris Prentiss. *The Book of Secrets: Unlocking the Hidden Dimensions of Your Life*, by Deepak Chopra, M.D., and *Zen-Brain Reflections*, by James Austin, M.D., provide information on the relationship of biofeedback 📖 and brain waves to Zen and hypnosis, plus comments on visual and auditory signals, mind-body music or art, and the medical usefulness of Zen. The Institute of Noetic Sciences (www.noetic.org) provides information on research into the potentials and powers of consciousness, including perceptions, beliefs, attention, intention, intuition, and parapsychology 📖. It explores phenomena that do not necessarily fit conventional scientific models, yet it maintains a commitment to scientific rigor.

What are some ways to improve your own sensory skills? The following sections in this chapter provide techniques and ideas. If you like, select some and use them frequently. You might like to use your personal notebook to record your impressions, thoughts, and results.

Observe with Concentration

Make a focused effort to use all of your five senses while blotting out conscious thought as thoroughly as possible. Just look at something common—a coin, a book—for a brief period of time, and focus on what you see. Now, while still looking at that object, focus on what is happening in the periphery. What are you aware of as your focus shifts? *Listen* to household sounds with your eyes closed, and concentrate on what you hear. *Touch* objects and hold them so that you really feel their shape, weight, texture, etc. *Look* with fresh eyes at clouds, your bedroom blinds, or your hand. *Taste* food, a small mouthful at a time, feel the sensations, and try to identify ingredients. Check familiar objects for odors, or get a bouquet of flowers and *smell* each separate blossom, noting how each is unique.

Sometimes you might want to consider the unusual properties of an object—the ones not quickly or easily noted. For example, in looking at a key, you may focus on its shape, surface color, and reflectivity while also recording mentally a lack of obvious odor. Contrary thinking, examining, and observing the extraordinary in the seemingly ordinary can yield interesting ideas.

Observe Repeatedly

Examine the same objects over a period of time, possibly under different circumstances. Note how changes in you—emotional or mental—may affect your sensations and how you begin to notice new aspects as time goes by. Seek a series of related events to observe for a prolonged period of time, perhaps months. People, weather, buildings, or certain landscapes are possibilities. Record these impressions on an ongoing basis.

Observe for a Purpose

As you collect observations, search for relationships within them. Make hypotheses about possible similarities, differences, cycles, patterns, and anomalies. Set up a schedule of observations designed to confirm or deny the expected relationships. Be careful. People tend, often unconsciously, to try to confirm first impressions. So strong is this tendency that you may ignore contradictory evidence. Use blinds or controls 📖 in order to minimize the likelihood that you are only confirming your initial beliefs.

Observe to Trigger Your Imagination

Investigate something and then mentally play with its essential characteristics. Imagine what would be necessary for it to be something else. How could it be similar to something that superficially appears to be very different? For example, there are many differences between a car and an orange, but how are they similar? Make your own pairings as ridiculous and extreme as possible. Then examine the objects and fantasize.

Alternatively, look at something, observe it, and try to imagine what it is like at levels beyond your ability to sense. You can sense the size, texture, color, and odor of a sheet of paper. But what lies beyond what you can see, feel, or smell? What does the paper release that you cannot observe? What inner structure is concealed? What equipment could you use to improve your observation?

Observe with Feedback

Sketch something that you have observed, and then compare your sketch with the actual object. You might use yourself, a pet, your room, your watch, etc. Some of these, such as your face, have emotional overtones that will affect your efforts considerably. The important thing here is not your artistic ability but your abstraction of reality as you see it. If you cannot draw, describe the object without naming it. Then ask someone to identify the object based solely on your written description.

Observe Yourself

This may be challenging but enjoyable. Ask yourself many questions, and then observe yourself. How long are your arms? How small an object can you see or feel? What sounds make you happy? How much food will you consume this week? How much peripheral vision do you have? In a room crowded with people, where would you choose to sit? How many words can you clearly speak in one minute? How far can you run in one minute? How much can you remember? What kinds of things do you remember? Can your fingertips distinguish between china and glass? These questions are just suggestions. Make up your own questions and find answers according to your interests.

Perhaps all of the emphasis on careful observation may seem like unnecessary effort to you. Yet observations such as these, made under complex conditions, have led to important ideas. In some of the afore-mentioned books on Zen, people learned to improve their health by controlling parts of their bodies that they thought were beyond their control. The results of this work have likely resulted in a decrease in premature deaths. Can you imagine what observations could have been designed by scientists to test ideas like this?

Precisely and carefully noticing any aspect of life is an essential step in understanding one's life. For example, your awareness of your body and its normal and abnormal conditions helps you determine your state of health and when to seek medical advice. Observation might enable you to use your body's sensory system in biofeedback techniques to help control tension or migraine headaches. Observing and evaluating body language can help you better understand friends and associates. A good test of this type of awareness is to turn it around and use it to imagine how others might see you. In all of these instances, you will be using your newly honed observational skills.

Finally, it is important for you to believe that you can see or sense something uniquely—whether for private pleasure and happiness, or possibly to discover something worth sharing with others. Don't wait for someone else to get you started by suggesting a project or something to examine. Find your own individual "child's eye" from which to observe the world.

Summary

- ▣ Situations and conditions affect your observational experiences.

- ▣ Your willingness to explore and observe is an inherent quality from childhood.

- ▣ Passive sensory information can stunt your observational growth.

- ▣ You should properly evaluate observations.

- ▣ Sensory efforts vary in intensity. Methods exist that can be used to increase this sensitivity.

- ▣ Different ways of practicing observing can sharpen your observation skills.

Words of Wisdom

Observation more than books, experience rather than persons, are the prime educators.
— Amos Bronson Alcott

All our knowledge begins with senses, proceeds then to understanding, and ends with reason.
— Immanuel Kant

To acquire knowledge, one must study; but to acquire wisdom, one must observe.
— Marilyn vos Savant

Minor things can become moments of great revelation when encountered for the first time.
— Margot Fonteyn

People who don't work with primary sources don't understand reality.
— Franklin Burroughs

What is a scientist after all? It is a curious man looking through a keyhole, the keyhole of nature, trying to know what's going on.
— Jacques Cousteau

That is what learning is. You should suddenly understand something you've understood all your life, but in a new way.
— Doris Lessing

Never get so fascinated by the extraordinary that you forget the ordinary.
— Magdalen Nabb

You can see a lot just by observing.
— Yogi Berra

We cannot create observers by just saying "observe," but by giving them the power and the means for this observation and these means are created through education of the senses.
– Maria Montessori

Opportunities are often things you haven't noticed the first time around.
– Catherine Deneuve

Chapter 4

Creative Thought Processes:
Activities to Increase Creativity

People who lovingly work with wood often say that each board is different—not just because one is pine and another is walnut, but because the grain pattern in each board is unique. The pattern tells the story of the tree's life. Did the sapling pine start out wedged between rocks? Was there a nearby overhanging wolf tree 📖 that limited the pine's growth because of the shadowed sun and shared root space? Did a storm cause a torn limb? Was there a bacterial attack? Did the wolf tree finally topple, allowing the pine to reach its crown out into an open sky? Each event shaped the pattern and texture of the wood.

Whereas a tree bears visible marks of its life experiences, people more often bear hidden recordings of their experiences. How? The way they think, their memory of history, their reaction to everyday events—all of these become their internal markings.

Your mobility, unique sensory system, and thinking ability make your process of living more complex than the pine tree. You see, feel, hear, imagine, construct, create, and travel through a web of unique personal experiences. This activity shapes and marks you as you seek favorable conditions for your growth and life.

For people who are creative, reaching toward personal expression within a culture is very much like the pine tree reaching toward sunlight. There is a common human need to use creativity to enliven and enhance daily life. As you seek your own personal expression, you may write, speak, or act creatively, and thus share and interpret life experiences. You may compare, rummage through a memory of words, seize a pen, and extend yourself into a cultural opening, like the pine tree reaching for the sky. These attempts to manage your own thoughts make you very special—a human being with creative possibilities.

Some human beings are limited by living narrowly, exposed to little outside experience of different people, places, or ideas. They are confined like the rock-bound pine. Some may feel overwhelmed by the abilities or activities of others and may be unable to reach out for their own share of "space" or recognition—like the pine in the shadow of the wolf tree. Some people have a physical disability or an illness that has left its mark. Yet it is important to remember that all life events can be handled positively, creatively, and as learning opportunities. As long as you live, you are a carrier of possibilities and an instrument of self-development—especially when you participate in life with a cheerful, open-minded attitude, ready to learn.

Most knowledge arrives via our senses, and people vary greatly in the sensitivity of their sensory thresholds or how well they use those senses. Some people have sensory disabilities and make use of aids such as eyeglasses or hearing aids which, coupled with creative thinking, help them achieve despite their handicap. For example, Beethoven 📖 contrived a way to feel vibrations from loudly played music that enabled him to continue composing music despite his deafness.

Whatever your sensory abilities, the more you expand your experiences and your ability to observe, the more likely you are to be able to think expansively and creatively. There is always something to find, observe, or create; immense opportunities exist for discovery.

But where do you find opportunities and challenges? Anywhere and everywhere! Creative thinking can involve making, fixing, or describing something. Thomas Edison's 📖 inventiveness—his most observable creative expression—often was in response to the changes in living conditions of his time. Out of the woven tapestry of everyday experiences, you too can isolate distinct questions, puzzles, or problems to solve.

Suppose you want to describe your home to a distant relative in a new and unusual way. You could consider using photographs, a written description, or a scale model. You begin thinking about how these portray your home. All of these methods depend primarily on sight, but your relative is blind. The scale model comes closest to being useful, because she could touch and feel it, but you think you can do something better. So you make an audio recording that portrays your passage through your house. The sounds include changes in your voice as well as in the sounds of footsteps on carpet versus vinyl, a radio playing, your younger brother crying—along with other descriptive comments, such as the number of steps taken in each room or your descriptions of items in each room. Instead of using the scale model, you developed a more original solution to your problem. Sometimes better solutions result when we diverge from traditional ideas.

Creativity requires thinking about things in new and different ways. When you think about a problem, use some fantasizing processes. Doodle pictures. Write a single sentence description. Ask questions. Why does this exist? When does this occur? Who needs this? Why? Then slide everything into your subconscious and let it incubate. Go to sleep. Listen to some music. Rest. Turn to other matters. Your subconscious may deliver a solution, perhaps even at 2:00 A.M. Be prepared with paper and pencil by your bedside. Many scientists and artists have gotten solutions to problems in this way.

Work at feeding your subconscious, continually and extensively. Experience everything deeply and widely, and you will increase your opportunities to be creative. For example, you might view Duchamp's painting, *Nude Descending a Staircase* 📖 and, without recognizing the source of inspiration, subsequently figure out a new and better way to guide blind people. While skiing, you might hear a particular sound effect as your skis swish rhythmically in the snow. Later, the sound becomes part of a musical passage—its source unidentified. Your background should be rich in "wild" or random information for future use. In addition, you need to know how to find and use information resources that are particular to your interests.

As Dr. Louis Pasteur said, "Chance favors the prepared mind." You need to be in good mental condition, always prepared to seize an elusive new idea.

Mental Conditioning

The following activities may help you keep in good mental condition. Try to use one or more of them regularly.

- ▣ Solve puzzles or mental games (charades, chess, Scrabble, crossword puzzles).

- ▣ Write short stories, poems, or music. Paint or sculpt.

◙ Maintain a creative interest in some special area. Attend relevant events.

◙ Carefully observe and describe something on a regular basis (faces, the sky, buildings, etc.).

◙ Imagine ways to improve situations around you. Note dissatisfaction with things as they are—cheerfully and creatively.

◙ Try to consider a question or problem of personal interest for 20 to 30 minutes without veering mentally.

◙ Try to find relationships between two very different objects. For example, pick an object and think of how it relates to some other object. This mental "doodling" usually begins with a thoughtful description of the objects. The most obvious properties will probably occur to you first. Search for similarities or differences that exist for these objects. Somewhere in this process, your background knowledge is being searched for congruent information relative to your descriptions. You continue to manipulate this information until there arises an "aha!" connection that is interesting, strange, or mentally arresting. A chain of thought develops with one idea producing another.

For example, consider a chair and a raisin—two very different objects—and the simplified chain of thought that is shown in the following sequence. Note when there is an "aha!" connection in this sample of one person's chain of thought.

Chair, wooden
Raisin, wrinkled
Wrinkles carved on a chair (Aha!)
Raisins
Raisin pie (Aunt Ella's)
Plump raisins
Raisin, grape
Grapevine, woody
Chair made of old grapevines (Aha!)
Grapes, picking
A chair device to pick grapes (Aha!)

This process uses divergent thinking. Notice that critical judgment is suspended. To practice this playful mental meandering, pick words as randomly as possible. Flip through a dictionary to choose words, or trade words with a challenging companion. This is a playful process, which may or may not yield any so-called "useful" ideas. The most important result is your increased awareness of the diversity in objects, your ability to think creatively, and possibly a developing awareness of looking more closely at your surroundings.

Use brainstorming techniques 📖 on a routine basis when you are attempting to solve problems. Record all ideas, as many as possible—the wild ones, the improbable ones, and the fit-together-with-something-else ones. Make no judgments as to value during this process. You might find checklists of words—such as those shown below which are designed to help creative thinking—useful in triggering your ideas for solutions. You may also want to try to develop your own checklist, similar to the "Possible Science Checklist" shown below, but specially suited to your area of interest and your experience. Use your personal notebook to record such checklists to use when you are faced with situations that particularly require creative thinking.

Possible General Checklist		Possible Science Checklist	
Substitute	Input	Optical	Alloy
Magnify	Shape	Electrical	Reaction
Minify	Time	Orientation	Specification
Reverse	Group	Tolerance	Function
Combine	Custom	Symmetry	Charge
Function	Place	Magnetic	Shape

For example, suppose you are writing a short story and cannot find a way to account for your hero's absence during a critical scene. You might use the "Possible General Checklist" to find alternate solutions, such as the ones that follow:

Substitute
He had to take his brother's place as an usher.

Magnify
He is in jail, accused of stealing.

Minify
Heedless of time, he is playing with his grandson.

Or perhaps for a science project you are to solve a problem of soil erosion. You might use the science checklist to creatively come up with some possible solutions.

Optical
Can I actually see greater erosion or changes in the dark colored soils?

Electrical
Do soil particle charges change after rainfall? Is this due to acidity?

Orientation
Is there a pattern of ridged surfaces?

Creative processes such as these can be used to solve problems or to discover or invent something new. One good idea may trigger two others, and a chain reaction ensues. Trading ideas in group sessions often can be more productive than working alone.

The opportunities to discover and know are nearly boundless, but they are seldom obvious or easy. If you do "walk into a wall," turn around and go the other way, or find a door, or poke a hole in the ceiling and grab a ladder. With practice and training, everyone can be more creative. Use your creativity. When you appreciate the vastness of the human imagination, become excited by the unknown, use all of your senses and abilities to explore, and share your creativity with others, you become beautifully marked by these efforts.

Summary

- Thinking processes are complex and personally unique.
- The extent of your related knowledge affects problem-solving processes.
- A subconscious "ripening" or incubation of a problem frequently produces answers.
- Creative efforts will almost surely make you more creative.
- Some specific procedures can be useful generators of ideas for problem-solving.
- A positive outlook improves chances for success in creative thinking.

Words of Wisdom

Imagination is the highest kite one can fly.
— Lauren Bacall

The shrewd guess, the fertile hypothesis, the courageous leap to a tentative conclusion—these are valuable coins of the thinker at work.
— Jerome Bruner

To walk on water, wait until it freezes.
— Jeffrey Woodruff Livingston

A problem is not solved in a laboratory. It is solved in some fellow's head, and all the apparatus is for is to get his head turned around so he can see the thing right.
— Charles F. Kettering

When a person never changes his mind, it's usually a pretty good indication that he's stopped thinking.
— Laura Van Wormer

To have ideas is to gather flowers; to think is to weave them into garlands.
— Anne Sophie Swetchine

If one is lucky, a solitary fantasy can totally transform one million realities.
— Maya Angelou

Our thought is the key, which unlocks the doors of the world.
— Samuel McChord Crothers

A rock pile ceases to be a rock pile the moment a single man contemplates it, bearing within him the image of a cathedral.
— Antoine de Saint-Exupéry

I like nonsense, it wakes up the brain cells. Fantasy is a necessary ingredient in living, it's a way of looking at life through the wrong end of a telescope. Which is what I do, and that enables you to laugh at life's realities.
– Dr. Theodore Geisel, a.k.a. Dr. Seuss

Think left and think right and think low and think high. Oh, the thinks you can think up if only you try.
– Dr. Theodore Geisel, a.k.a. Dr. Seuss

Creativity represents a miraculous coming together of the uninhibited energy of the child with its apparent opposite and enemy, the sense of order imposed on the disciplined adult intelligence.
– Norman Podhoretz

Trust that little voice in your head that says "Wouldn't it be interesting if..." And then do it.
– Duane Michals

The most beautiful thing we can experience is the mysterious. It is the source of all true art and science. He to whom the emotion is a stranger, who can no longer pause and stand wrapped in awe, is as good as dead; his eyes are closed.
– Albert Einstein

The creative person is both more primitive and more cultivated, more destructive, a lot madder and a lot saner, than the average person.
– Frank Barron

Chapter 5

Speed Reading: A Vital Key

Reading is an intellectual art, a canvassing of human thought, and a crucial tool in shaping your life. If you read successfully, you can quickly recognize letter and word patterns, and you will associate them with personal experiences. This produces mental images and ideas. If you are not able to read clearly and quickly, you may avoid the act of reading altogether and thus miss the joys—not to mention the knowledge—that can come from reading.

Reading rapidly is desirable, but reading faster and remembering less is traveling in the wrong direction. Therefore, speed reading means reading as fast as possible, considering your ability and the type of material, while retaining enough to have made the reading worthwhile. If you have not already learned this, it should be a relief to learn that good readers seldom read every word; this is one way to increase your reading rate.

You can develop and use different strategies for a variety of reading purposes. For example, you won't read a science book the same way you read the sports page in the newspaper. For the science book, you might first scan all of the headings and bold print words to become familiar with key concepts. Then you might skim each section quickly for an overview of ideas. Finally, you will go back to more thoroughly read each section for understanding. For the sports page, you will likely read quickly and then may stop after the second line. You may only need to know how a certain player scored. You read, looking for the score, and then turn the page.

Always consider your purpose for reading and the amount of time you have available. President Kennedy allowed himself only a half an hour to skim through three newspapers every morning at breakfast. With limited time, he still wanted to scan the headlines and relevant articles. Whatever the purpose for your reading, learning and practicing speed reading techniques will allow you to read and retain more material. You will be able to double, and in some cases triple, your reading speed and comprehension from what it is now if you practice using some of the techniques described in this chapter.

Some helpful suggestions for reading improvement follow.

Physical Conditions

- Make sure that vision problems have been corrected to the best extent possible; have regular eye examinations.

- Choose reading surroundings that are quiet and not intrusive.

- Use lighting that minimizes glare.

- Set up your reading area with paper, pens, pencils, a dictionary, and any other needed materials.

- If the reading is very demanding, take a five-minute break every half-hour. Walk around, look at distant objects, close your eyes, listen to some music, or do a minor chore.

- Sit in a chair that provides good back support and does not promote sleepiness.

Eye Span and Return Sweeps

Do you know how to increase efficiency by increasing your reading eye span? Your present eye span may only allow you to see one or two medium-length words of average type size at a time. With a little practice, you can enlarge your eye span to look at four or five words at a time. Make a slotted card that can frame typical three- to four-word lengths. By sliding it along, you can become accustomed to viewing a longer line of type on the page.

Going from one-word recognition to three-word recognition more than triples your reading comprehension speed. Why? The cluster of words can produce ideas and images that are more complex and meaningful. For example, consider your responses sequentially to the following: *bright*, then *bright blue*, then finally, *bright blue balloon.* If each word is responded to singly, the mind "clutters" with unnecessary images, and reading is slowed as a result. "Chunking" improves the speed of information sent to the brain.

You can also improve return eye sweeps. These occur when the eyes move from the end of one line to the beginning of the next. Slow or inaccurate sweeps decrease speed. One simple way to improve sweep is to hold a piece of paper under each line, allowing you to only see one line at a time. When you finish the line, move the paper down. This will help train your eyes to sweep correctly across to the next line. An alternate activity to increase reading speed is to hold a piece of paper above each line, and then to increase the rate at which you move the paper down the page.

Other rapid reading techniques using eye-hand coordination are described in *Speed Reading: The Easy Way* by Howard Stephen Berg and Marcus Conyers. They show that it is possible to increase reading rate from 200 words per minute to at least 2,000 words per minute. Another excellent book with many practical techniques is *Breakthrough Rapid Reading* by Peter Kump.

Improving and Expanding Your Vocabulary

If you have a small vocabulary, your reading is impeded. You must either skip each unknown word, with potential loss of meaning, or stop to check it in a dictionary. Here are some suggestions for improving and expanding your vocabulary:

- Obtain a dictionary.

- In your personal notebook, begin a list of new vocabulary words from your readings.

- Make homemade flash cards with the new word on one side and the definition on the other side. (Also, note the pronunciation.) Flip through these cards once or twice a week.

- Try to incorporate your new words into your conversations and writing.

Visualization

"Think while you read" in order to turn printed ideas into vivid personal pictures. Think of exciting stories you have read in the past and the pictures of all the characters you created in your mind's eye. Do you remember Winnie the Pooh or Harry Potter? Those characters are easy to recall, and the stories were easy to read because of visual pictures you created in your mind.

Do the same sort of picture imaging with all of your reading. Associate technical or more difficult words with other terms that can be transformed into pictures. If you are reading about something so foreign to you that images cannot be formed, obtain supplemental material. For example, when reading about Medieval Europe and the Knights of the Round Table 📖, you might find a book with illustrations of typical castle architecture helpful.

Reading improvement also occurs if you can decrease vocalization (sounding out words half-aloud or forming words with your lips) and instead concentrate only on sight-reading. This is a much quicker way to read but requires that you practice keeping your lips still.

Another reading shortcut comes from developing quick visual familiarity with the style and content of the material before reading it thoroughly. For example, prefaces and other introductory materials often provide information about the overall framework, as well as the writer's purpose and point of view—all essential to your understanding of your reading. Very experienced rapid readers scan for key words or focus their sight on the centers of paragraphs. Then, they either visually reject the surplus words or note them peripherally. This can be risky, however, especially with technical material. Initially, this style of reading is difficult, but its mastery can be useful where precise awareness of content is not necessary, such as in reading fiction.

Mnemonics

Since reading depends so much upon memory, memory aids can enhance your reading skills. You can create a pattern or system to help you remember the new material. You might remember an unusual term because it sounds like something else with which you are more familiar (e.g., hone and bone), has a similar beginning to a related word (e.g., mnemonics, memory), or has a recognizable form in another language (e.g., prisoner, prisonier). Eventually it will be mentally simpler and more efficient to have direct recall of a term's meaning, but using a mnemonic scheme can help at the outset. As a suggestion, obtain a book on memory or mnemonics or look up this topic on the Internet, and try some of the exercises.

Paper and Pen Reading

When you read, keep a pen or pencil handy to make notes. Gilbert Keith Chesterton 📖 and Georg Bernard Shaw 📖 maintained an unusual correspondence with each other by exchanging books that they annotated in the margins. Their comments were often peppery because of their conflicting philosophies. This type of correspondence became practical only because they personally owned the books they used to mentally challenge each other.

If you own a book that has limited value, such as a paperback or used book, you may want to underline or use a yellow marker to highlight key ideas. You may want to make additional marginal notations for review purposes.

If you don't own the book that you are reading or if you don't like to write directly in your books, you may want to use notebooks, file cards, or a computer to record valuable ideas or to make comments about the content. You could also write comments on "sticky notes" and place them on the actual page.

Paper and pen reading has a number of benefits. The physical activity of writing actually helps keep your mind alert. Also, "smart laziness," or efficiency, ensues. Condensing 100 words of original content to just a sentence or a five-word phrase may make an important idea more memorable.

As you read, ask yourself questions. What do I know about this? What should I know? Why does the author say this? Do I agree with the author? Why or why not? Asking questions as you read makes the reading go easier and faster, and you will remember better what you read. This questioning technique also improves your understanding of the relevance of the content to your life.

Practice

Reading, like any other skill, improves with practice. Reading requires repetitive experiences to reach satisfactory performance levels, especially if you are a poor reader. To improve, you should set aside time for practice. Some of your reading will be for knowledge and perspective, but some should simply be for pleasure. Choose your reading material wisely by considering possible returns for time spent, and consciously use the ideas listed above to increase your speed.

Selection and Material

Select material that really interests you and has reasonable print size. The writing should have a style and vocabulary that is slightly challenging but not overwhelming. Obtain suggestions for your reading from knowledgeable friends, librarians, bibliographies, and book reviews. Use the Internet to search for books on a topic, and look for reviews of books on sites such as Amazon.com. Go to a library and browse through the new books display, or look in the stacks at books in areas that are unknown to you; read book jackets, and leaf through randomly selected passages. If you have always read mysteries or science fiction, consider expanding your reading interests to include biography or history.

Life Experience

A reader with limited life experience often finds it difficult to understand the significance of what is being read. Of course, we do broaden our life experience through reading, but such experience is second-hand and often lacks depth and perspective. There is no simple solution to this problem. By acquiring first-hand diverse experience at every opportunity, you will broaden your base of understanding. Whatever your extent of life experience, the most important thing is that your mind is thinking and processing as you read.

Summary

To improve reading skills:

- Check physical conditions such as lighting.
- Increase your eye span, improve eye sweeps, and use scanning.
- Expand your vocabulary; turn printed words into pictures in your mind's eye.
- Decrease or eliminate vocalization; avoid reading "half-aloud."
- Use mnemonics or other memory aids.
- As you read, ask questions about content to increase your understanding of relevance and to enhance your memory.
- Set aside time to practice reading, and choose wisely what you read.
- Expand your own personal life experiences.

Words of Wisdom

Some books are to be tasted, others to be swallowed, and some few to be chewed and digested: that is, some books are to be read only in parts, others to be read, but not curiously, and some few to be read wholly, and with diligence and attention.
— Francis Bacon

Just the knowledge that a good book is awaiting one at the end of a long day makes that day happier.
— Kathleen Norris

The big advantage of a book is it's very easy to rewind. Close it and you're right back at the beginning.
— Jerry Seinfeld

Reading without reflecting is like eating without digesting.
— Edmund Burke

If we encountered a man of rare intellect, we should ask him what books he read.
— Ralph Waldo Emerson

The greatest gift is the passion for reading. It is cheap, it consoles, it distracts, it excites, it gives you knowledge of the world and experience of a wide kind. It is a moral illumination.
— Elizabeth Hardwick

Reading furnishes our mind only with materials of knowledge; it is thinking that makes what we read ours.
— John Locke

You can think your pain and heartbreak are unprecedented in the history of the world, but then you read. It was books that taught me that the things that tormented me most were the very things that connected me with all the people who were alive, or who had ever been alive.
– James Baldwin

I took a speed reading course and read War and Peace in twenty minutes. It involves Russia.
– Woody Allen.

I am not a speed reader. I am a speed understander.
– Isaac Asimov

A wonderful thing about a book, in contrast to a computer screen, is that you can take it to bed with you.
– Daniel J. Boorstin

Never judge a book by its movie.
– J. W. Eagan

I suggest that the only books that influence us are those for which we are ready, and which have gone a little farther down our particular path than we have yet got ourselves.
– E. M. Forster

Surviving and thriving as a professional today demands two new approaches to the written word. First, it requires a new approach to orchestrating information, by skillfully choosing what to read and what to ignore. Second, it requires a new approach to integrating information, by reading faster and with greater comprehension.
– Jimmy Calano

Chapter 6

Enthusiasm and Confidence: Impressive and Infectious

The world is full of avenues for exploration. For example, you may have discovered the richness of the American art pottery movement, or the challenges of painting miniatures, or an unusual musical toccata. Perhaps you have invented a new product, or you see a way to solve a community problem. Enthusiastically, you share your excitement with everyone. Sometimes, however, you get rebuffed and thus discover one of the few drawbacks of being really excited about anything.

But suppose one day you decide that you have proceeded far enough with an idea to seek advice from several experts. The first expert praises your scholarship, intuition, and discoveries. The second points out some problems, errors in judgment, and flaws in reasoning. When you think about these conflicting opinions, you see new ways to approach your topic. After talking with these authorities, you have even more confidence in your work, are no longer hesitant, and remain enthusiastic. The first expert's encouraging words prevented you from giving up too soon when your work became difficult. The second expert's critique helped you develop needed changes. Most importantly, you retained your confidence and self-esteem throughout this process, which allowed you to also retain your enthusiasm and creative effort.

Enthusiasm and Well-Being

Having enthusiasm is an important part of your well-being. Observe people you know. Which ones are absorbed in an interest? What effect does this excitement have upon their life? As you study the lives of famous people through biographies and autobiographies, does their enthusiasm seem obvious? Are their hobbies, talents, community involvement, or career efforts central to that person's lifestyle? For example, Franklin D. Roosevelt 📖 was an avid stamp collector. Thomas Jefferson 📖 had many strong interests, including architecture and gardening. Hobbies not only enrich your leisure time, but they also may develop into full-time careers later. Among the people you know, are there any who have hobbies? Contrast their lives with those who do not. What do you conclude?

Whether your enthusiasm is toward a hobby or some other endeavor, enthusiasm provides power for your interests. Under the right circumstances, enthusiasm is contagious and can motivate groups. How do you get enthusiasm? Some people seem only to catch second-hand enthusiasms; they never start their own. They attend popular events, seek occupations that have crowd approval, and read magazines and newspapers to determine what they like. They wear clothing with labels as status symbols to bolster their confidence. Others have enthusiasm generated from within. They plan events that excite them, follow their personal interests, and are happy with themselves. Try to have that kind of enthusiasm.

Self-Generated Enthusiasm

To nurture your own self-generated enthusiasm, let your self emerge without listening to the voices of parents, authority, tradition, the experts, or the status-seekers. Stay as close as possible to your own inner world. Believe in fresh sight, and accept the possibility that reasoning can be flawed and that facts can be added to, changed, and rearranged. Transcend the limitations that reason and tradition are always trying to impose. Would you describe Picasso 📖 as being a "second-hand enthusiast"? With his prodigious output, his innovative adventuring, and his hearty enjoyment of life, "primogenitor enthusiast" is a better label.

Primogenitor, or self-generated, enthusiasm requires intensive efforts of introspection, self-discovery, and self-development. Look at the enthusiasm and confidence of salespeople who depend upon their belief in themselves, their product line, and their ability to understand their customers to do their job well. The skill of relating to people is the art of successful sales. Good salespeople are creative. Supersalesman Joe Girard 📖 shares many of his sales techniques in several books worth reading.

Some people experience a drive toward reaching their personal potential. These persons have "peak" experiences, or what the psychologist Csikszentmihalyi calls the "flow" of optimal experiences. Often these individuals are so enthusiastic and involved in their projects that they lose track of time and place. It is personally gratifying to realize one's capabilities and then to understand that it is possible to develop most, if not all, of those capabilities.

Nurturing Enthusiasm

But how do you nurture and maintain enthusiasm once your initial response dwindles? Your failure to be enthusiastic may occur because certain activities are no longer enlightening or give you intellectual stimulation. Even when everything is bleakest and darkest, you can find resources within or without that can rekindle the excitement. For example, suppose you have always enjoyed cryptography 📖. But lately, you find it a dead-end, no longer challenging or fun. Yet you really do not wish to let it go; some part of you is still attached and interested. Perhaps you can add cryptography to something else in order to create a new interest. For example, combine it with literature to write a novel or detective story, or use a page in your notebook to brainstorm other combinations. If you are certain that your love affair with codes is over, it is probably time for you to find something new and to turn your attention elsewhere.

Beware of being the dilettante enthusiast—quick to embrace and quick to reject items to explore. Allow your interests to consume you for a significant period of time. Otherwise, you may never experience "seeing below the surface" and are far less likely to be an innovator.

At the other extreme, you might be tempted to hold on to your interest and enthusiasm beyond the point of reasonableness. When it approaches the comfortableness of an old shoe, it is time to go shopping for a new area of interest. Gerald M. Loeb 📖, a brilliant stock market investor, used a formula to cut his market losses to a minimum. He applied the ratchet effect (a ratchet prevents reversal of motion); when his investments *began* to slip backward, he froze his gains and got out of the market. The same principle can be used for investments of self and time. When something begins to pall, give it critical examination and consider applying a ratchet.

But what about tasks in front of you, particularly if they are unchosen, unloved, and uninteresting? Can you summon enthusiasm for things you do not care about? Why not? If you can regard enthusiasm as a feasible alternative to boredom, hatred, or distaste, you will have the beginning of a good solution to such mundane tasks. Use your creative wit. Dream up excitement. Find relationships between the present situation and something you care about. Fantasize. Construct images. Regard the present as an opportunity to observe accurately. However, if even with your best effort some matters cannot be greeted enthusiastically, so be it.

Your enthusiasms should be selective. If you are enthusiastic about everything, enthusiasms fail to please and inform. Contrast in your life between blandness and excitement is essential. As long as something excites you, storms your entire being, and holds you enthralled, all is well.

One special kind of enthusiasm can totally engulf you. It is the zeal associated with a cause. The etymology of "enthusiasm" is based on Greek terms meaning divinely inspired; all of that archaic meaning is related to religious emotions and inspirations. Modern causes may or may not have religious origins, but they are sources of enthusiasm nonetheless. Some popular causes include environmental issues, racial and social discrimination, animal rights, rebuilding of cities, and saving historical landmarks. Find a cause that suits you and your available time. Work at it. You will meet people, gain valuable skills, and feel good inside. You may even find your life's work developing from this cause. Even better, choose a cause that is associated with your career interests.

When It's Hard to Be Enthusiastic

What about "down days" when you find it hard to be enthusiastic about things that are usually pleasurable? When the effort to enjoy doing pleasant tasks is difficult, remember that everyone has "down days." Assuming that you are not physically tired (perhaps from lack of sleep—then take a nap), the best advice is to get busy, take a brisk walk, clean your desk, or make something. One young man solved this problem in a unique way. He kept the ingredients for homemade chili on hand and made a large batch whenever "down days" occurred. Then he called friends and invited them to come and dine. By reaching out and becoming involved in the outside world, he was able to overcome the blankness or emptiness of these occasional days.

What if your "down days" are more than occasional? You may be suffering from depression, a condition that can be relieved by medical or psychological attention. Talk to your family or friends. Get help from your family doctor. Sometimes professional help is needed to regain your interests and be enthusiastic again. Then, once more, you will be able to trust your ability to assess events realistically, to find satisfaction in using your ability, and to take pleasure in being creative.

Sharing Your Enthusiasm

Our society does not grant nor refuse the right to be enthusiastic. You can pick your "thing" just about as freely as you can pick flowers in spring. But you may not have as much freedom in gaining societal respect and support for your enthusiasms. Here are some valuable tips:

- Ideas are more quickly accepted from people who fit certain patterns of behavior and appearance—those who have the "right image" or the "right stuff." This is not to say that you should change who you are, but be aware that people may not hear a message because they are distracted by the messenger. Sometimes fitting in with a society is the best way to infiltrate new ideas.

- Sometimes new ideas are opposed by others simply because they challenge the tradition and the status quo. Is it possible to change this regrettable circumstance? Yes. History is rife with societies resisting changes that have been introduced by creative people, particularly if these persons were women, minorities, renegade artists, and political dissidents. Yet these individuals used their determined persistence, persuasiveness, and enthusiasm to eventually overwhelm the opposition. Can you persist? You may want to investigate all possible avenues of publicity to keep your cause alive. You could write letters and articles, meet influential people, join organizations, use the Internet, organize public events—all hard work. Strong enthusiasm is worth effort. Great enthusiasm is worth exceptional effort.

◪ Your interests and enthusiasms describe and measure you. They tell your size—not in feet or pounds but in feats and sounds. Out of all possible interests, what have you chosen and why? What have you done with your choice? Have you confined your passion to a private sanctum, or have you shared it? What deeds, songs, or sayings have you set forth?

Have you managed to make your life a network of enthusiasms? Do these touch other humans in accord with eternal verities such as truth, beauty, kindness, and all the other finest ideals of human conception? If they do, your enthusiasm will bring you self-confidence and assurance that is impressive and infectious.

Summary

◪ Sharing enthusiasms is a risky but essential and rewarding process.

◪ Some enthusiasms arise from popular sources; others arise from personal effort.

◪ Self-generated enthusiasms develop in response to intense self-search and open-mindedness.

◪ Enthusiasms can be short-lived, humdrum, or exchanged.

◪ Causes can provide unusual inspiration.

◪ Pursued enthusiasms yield confidence.

Words of Wisdom

If you are all wrapped up in yourself, you are overdressed.
— Kate Halverson

If you wish in this world to advance
Your merits you're bound to enhance;
You must stir it and stump it,
And blow your own trumpet,
Or, trust me, you haven't a chance.
— W. S. Gilbert

You grow up the day you have your first real laugh at yourself.
— Ethel Barrymore

Somehow, I can't believe that there are any heights that can't be scaled by a man who knows the secret of making dreams come true. This special secret, it seems to me, can be summarized in four C's. They are curiosity, confidence, courage, and constancy, and the greatest of these is confidence. When you believe in a thing, believe in it all the way, implicitly and unquestionably.
— Walt Disney

Confidence comes not from always being right but from not fearing to be wrong.
— Peter T. McIntyre

There is real magic in enthusiasm…. It gives warmth and good feeling to all your personal relationships.
— Norman Vincent Peale

Nothing great was ever achieved without enthusiasm.
— Ralph Waldo Emerson

Self-confidence is the first requisite to great undertakings.
— Samuel Johnson

You have to have confidence in your ability, and then be tough enough to follow through.
— Rosalynn Carter

Ability is what you're capable of doing. Motivation determines what you do. Attitude determines how well you do it.
— Lou Holtz

I am afraid to show you who I really am, because if I show you who I really am, you might not like it—and that's all I got.
— Sabrina Ward Harrison

Often the difference between a successful person and a failure is not that one has better abilities or ideas, but the courage that one has to bet on one's ideas , to take a calculated risk—and to act.
— Andre Malraux

Chapter 7

Decision Making: Five Steps to Making Wise Choices

Suppose you are attending a party that has become boring. You consider your options:

- Leaving.

- Figuring out how you can add some excitement.

- Getting someone else to join with you to make it more interesting.

- Inciting someone else to "make it more lively."

Which is the right choice? Which would you choose? There might be alternative solutions, but there is no "right" answer to the party problem. This is true of most other problems or situations requiring decisions as well. You make your decision based on choices that are in line with your personal beliefs and values, your knowledge, cultural experiences, interests, and personality. Sometimes a decision is made out of habit (e.g., "I've always done it that way"), and sometimes people avoid making a decision at all, which is its own kind of decision. Making the decision not to decide keeps the issue in limbo or allows others to step in and make the decision for you, which may not be what you want. Hopefully, though, most of your decisions will be active and thoughtful ones. And like other abilities, your decision-making skills will improve with practice.

You Are the Constant in Your Decisions

Throughout your efforts to reach any decision, there will be one constant presence—you, with all of your various experiences and your personality. Using the same information, events, and circumstances, would someone else arrive at the same decision as you? Possibly. Possibly not. For example, a journalist narrowly escapes being killed in a building collapse. The differences between the descriptions of various eyewitnesses concerning that event are more apparent to him now because he was directly involved in the situation himself, and his account is not the same as many of the others. As a result of this dramatic event, he decides to change his style of reporting to rely less on eyewitness accounts and more on solid facts. This reporter's experience and knowledge, derived from this one incident, also influences his decision to write more investigative pieces in the future. Eventually, he uses his new fact-finding skills to write articles that contribute to the revision of regulations governing the local construction industry. Do you think you would have been affected in the same way by this experience? Will events in your life affect your future decision making?

The way you view life and customarily respond to events and experiences also influences your decisions. Are you future-oriented? Can you look beyond today and consider both the short-term and long-term consequences of a decision you are contemplating? Are you capable of making good decisions that run counter to common expectations? What is your balance between undertaking a calculated risk and being foolhardy? Your personality is showing!

Your personality certainly contributes to your style of decision making. Recall the party scenario from the beginning of this chapter. Which action would you choose? Are you shy or introverted? If so, you might decide to leave the dull party. Are you an instigator? Then you might decide to get someone else to start a new game or activity. Are you a socializer or good at sharing? Perhaps you and a friend could put on a great act. Your personality will influence the manner with which you approach a choice.

Decisions are also based on information, either spoken or written. But it is important to realize that information often can be inaccurately perceived. You need to be sensitive to tone of voice, customary verbal style, and body language in order to evaluate communications that could affect your decisions. Even with the best of intentions, people do not always mean what they say.

Rude people and other disagreeable personalities can also influence your decisions, sometimes irritating you so much that you may not want to respond to their requests or accept needed information from them. For instance, while at work, a coworker may rudely ask you to do something that needs to be finished. You might find yourself tempted to ignore this request simply because of the way in which your coworker asked you to do it. However, not completing this task may cause both you and your coworker to be fired, which is certainly detrimental to you. Instead, try to concentrate on solving problems in a way that is most beneficial to you and least harmful (perhaps even beneficial) to those who tend to offend. Getting caught up in emotional reactions to other people can limit your vision and lead to poor choices.

Factors that Favor Good Decisions

Before approaching any decision, you may want to think about factors that favor making good decisions. This list includes your ability to:

- Know and care about yourself and others.

- Sense opportunities within changing conditions.

- Keep an optimistic view of the future.

- Identify and accept good ideas, valid information, and advice.

- Develop many and diverse ideas.

- Tolerate others who are different from you, and learn from them.

- Be aware of your feelings and values.

- Believe in the goodness within you and others.

- Accept responsibility with mature assurance.

- Benefit from failure by learning how to succeed next time.

Few people can be all of the above even some of the time. But just being conscious of these ideas and attempting to include them in your approach to decisions can still make a significant difference in the end result. Perhaps you think you are too young or too powerless to make a difference by your decisions. In fact, however, the most innovative changes in society have been spawned by youth. The need for good decisions has never been exhausted, and there will always be a need for them.

Some decisions are difficult; others are easy and almost automatic. Your everyday decisions usually are not made with much forethought. Frequently, you act out of habit when you greet people, choose food, or fill a coffee cup for a friend. Some of these decisions may seem trivial. However, there are consequences for all acts. A pleasant greeting tends to attract people to you—a basis for developing friendships. Good eating habits tend to keep you healthy. Some habits may not be beneficial. The decision to smoke could lead to an addiction, which could result years later in painful death from lung cancer or emphysema. A review of your everyday habitual decisions can be revealing and helpful.

Other types of decisions allow a more leisurely approach, permitting you to gather facts and information before you decide and to use some creative thinking processes as you examine your options. A decision about whether to enter a contest or apply for a new job will require some time for gathering and analyzing data. One quick strategy for reviewing information in this type of decision making is simply to list the pros and cons of the decision in two columns on a sheet of paper. When you are finished, compare the lists and make your decision.

Most people have trouble making major decisions. What is a decision facing you now or in the future? Why is this decision important? What sort of process will you use to help you decide? Will it be random, or will it be deliberate and thoughtful? Think back on a good decision you have made. Why was it good? Think back to a poor decision you have made. What made it a poor decision?

Five Stages in Decision Making

The initiating force behind every decision is change. Changes in your life lead to the need for decisions—sometimes simple, sometimes complicated. Being able to sense changes as soon as they occur may help you develop unique and creative responses of lasting value.

There are five basic stages to thoughtful decision making. Let's set up an example of how to use these stages to arrive at a good decision. Assume that you have a car that is older and continually breaking down. You'd like to buy a newer car, but then you'd have to get a loan and make regular monthly payments. A relative in your family gave you your current car, so you aren't used to that monthly burden. You can't decide if it would be better to keep your old car since you don't have a loan on it, but it keeps costing you money in repairs, or if it would be advisable to purchase a newer car and make a monthly financial commitment which you aren't used to doing.

Using the following system can be quite helpful in making this and other difficult decisions.

Stage 1: Define the Problem

The first stage of decision making is understanding problems and opportunities, and it is made up of a seemingly disconnected series of questions and reactions. Why is this happening now? How is this possible? What is involved? When do I have to act? This process is actually a preliminary defining of the problem by including an awareness of what it is, narrowing its dimensions, and realizing how it affects you and others.

Often it is essential to accurately identify the issue at hand before you attempt any further efforts. Wisely, you should also match your effort to the size and seriousness of the problem. To start the more complete process of defining, make a list of what you believe is the nature of the issue. Use as many as possible of the following "describers" to assist you in this process.

- What has (or has not) happened that makes a decision necessary?
- Who has (or has not) changed in this situation?
- When did (or will) this situation occur?
- Where did (or does) this happen?
- Why is this a problem (or opportunity)?
- Do I have the authority to make a decision?
- Do I have the means to act if I make a decision?
- How quickly do I have to make a decision?
- What information or assistance do I need?

Try to divide a complicated situation into smaller pieces before using the "describers." For our example, you should first investigate how much work your current car is likely to need in the near future. Perhaps you should check out what the price range is for quality used cars that you might like to own. You may also want to see if you qualify for financing if you do decide to purchase a newer vehicle. Now imagine how the "describers" might be utilized through each part of this problem.

As you use the "describers" to sort out information on the issue of your car (or any issue that you are dealing with), write out a list of answers. Perhaps the answers seem sketchy, but remember, they can provide important structure for future action. By using the answers, you can create a timeframe and realize your needs concerning this issue. This defining has another benefit—it keeps you active, focused, and moves the process along. If you have the flexibility, allow the problem to "rest" for a few days while you gather conscious (and subconscious) ideas and information.

Collecting practical knowledge is essential in defining, as it is throughout all the stages of working on a decision. A mistake often made by decision makers is not using something because they aren't aware that it exists. For example, maybe you believe that you cannot get financing for a new vehicle, but you are unaware that you could qualify if you had a co-signer on the loan, which is something that your parents might agree to do. Information from other people can help you understand the nature and dimension of a problem that you are trying to define—especially when different ideas are shared freely in an atmosphere of mutual trust and respect. Your willingness to seek and use valid information from many sources makes you a better, more confident decision maker.

Stage 2: Setting a Goal

After working with the "describers" and defining the problem or opportunity, what's next? What do you want to do about this issue? You need to select a specific goal, aim, or target if you are to attain a solution. This is stage two of the decision-making process.

Perhaps you have heard the saying, "If you don't know where you're going, any road will take you there." Setting goals is a way of getting things moving in the right direction. One of the best methods for achieving goals later is to write them down now. Once you have established that you want to do something, your mind can begin planning how best to make it happen, even subconsciously. If you write that you want to have a newer car sometime before you go off to college so that you won't have to worry about getting there and back, then your mind can now begin thinking and planning for that goal.

You may find that many different goals are involved in helping you reach your final decision. Perhaps you will have to get a higher paying job in order to purchase a newer car. However, maybe you have been looking at better jobs that are more oriented toward what you would like to do for a career. Your problem with your car may in fact be the catalyst for helping you achieve a better career opportunity. In most cases, good decisions favor the coincidence of reaching many goals.

In general, goals tend to fit into two categories—broadly encompassing and narrowly specific. A broadly encompassing goal might be to seek ways to enhance your happiness, select a career, or choose a mate. A narrowly specific goal could include completing a list of telephone calls you need to make by a certain date. Goals that merit the most serious consideration are those that could have a prolonged influence in the future upon you and others. However, life does not ensure the accuracy of predictions. Therefore, the wise person remains alert to changing conditions and thoughtfully adjusts goals accordingly.

Stage 3: Hypothesize Solutions

The considerations of goals and the future are the background for the third stage in the decision-making process. You have already defined your problem or opportunity and have set goals. It is time to hypothesize in order to figure out potential solutions. After defining the issue and giving it time to "rest," perhaps you came up with some ideas. Begin by listing your ideas in your personal notebook, on a computer, or on a wall chart.

You may need to use some devices to nourish your imagination. Some people schedule creative thinking time and listen to music, while others need total quiet. Flipping through books or magazines or surfing the Internet can help spark ideas. You may find that creative ideas can be triggered by visual information contained in illustrations on unrelated topics. For example, you may be looking at a picture of a winter river scene on a wall at the doctor's office, and your mind wanders off to the song lyrics "over the river and through the woods to grandmother's house we go." This may spark the memory that your grandmother told you several months ago that she'd like her garage painted. She even offered to pay you. Perhaps you could do this and other chores for other family members in order to come up with money for a down payment on a car.

Ideas arrive like fireflies from the darkness of night. Enlightenment can occur suddenly, or it can elude you for days. Patience is an ally. Keep gathering information relative to your problem. Record all of your ideas—without judgment—until you have obtained a number of solutions that seem reasonable.

Stage 4: Judgment by Ranking

When you seem to have reached the limit of potential solutions, or when you are driven by time constraints, you have reached the fourth stage—judgment. You begin this stage by ranking your potential solutions according to how useful they are to you. In this preliminary sequence, you will be responding to a complex collection of personal values, emotions, intuition, knowledge, and experience. When your list is finished, take your first choice and check its usefulness by questioning how well it solves all aspects of the described situation. This examination may cause you to rearrange your ranking. For this evaluation, the following checklist (which particularly applies to creative effort) may be helpful.

- Is the amount of effort required reasonable?

- Is the amount of needed material or equipment practical?

- Will it produce timely results?

- Is it reversible? Can anything else be done if it doesn't work?

- Is it likely to produce new or unusually good results?

- Is it likely that you can get the needed equipment, money, publicity, etc.?

- Is it of low or high risk?

- Are there likely to be negative consequences?

- Is it likely to produce fewer problems than it solves?

- Is it likely to be useful in solving other problems or in creating other opportunities?

- Is it legal, moral, and ethical?

- Is it culturally acceptable, and how much do you care if it is not?

You may wish to develop other checklists to help you in solving interpersonal or other specific problems. Use your checklist to evaluate the potential solutions, keeping in mind the possibility that you may already have a preconceived idea or even a personal bias. For example, maybe you really want a new car so badly that you aren't honestly evaluating your potential solutions for how best to keep your old one running for a few more years, which may be the most practical solution for you at the present time. When possible, you might seek a second opinion or even feedback from a group of evaluators. What you are developing is a narrowing list of options.

You will probably develop a style of selection and, if successful, you will keep it. For example, one style might give first choice to the option that could produce a large payoff with little effort—even though it is an outside chance or long shot. Another style would make as your choice of last resort any selection that is irreversible. Review your decisions (and your style of decision making) on separate occasions, with some intervening time for reflection. Two good questions to ask yourself are:

1. What will be the first result of this option?

2. What will be the lasting result of this option?

Sometimes, you may find yourself feeling stressed about the possible outcomes of your decisions. Often it helps to consider the possible outcomes in three ways. That is, what would be: (a) the absolute worst outcome, (b) the best possible result, and (c) the most likely consequence. Think about these three, and look for evidence as to which outcome is most likely. You might also wish to write down your predictions to be reviewed at a later time. You may want to read *The Resilience Factor: 7 Keys to Finding Your Inner Strenth and Overcoming Life's Hurdles*, by the psychologists Reivich and Shatté, who describe how this approach to decision making can reduce stress and enhance your own personal resilience.

Hopefully, your reflection will help you avoid using unwise decision-making processes. Some particular examples of foolish or careless decision-making approaches would include:

- I'll toss a coin.
- I'll do it the usual way; it has always worked.
- I'll jump right in before someone else does.
- I'll hope no one notices.
- I'll just do this; there is no other way.
- I'll try anything; something is bound to work.
- I'll do nothing and hope the problem goes away.

Stage 5: Making the Decision

As the number of options dwindle to only a few equally acceptable possibilities, you have arrived at the final, or fifth, stage—the decision itself, with perhaps an alternate choice. The final selection is made by reviewing all of your knowledge of the present situation, while considering experience with previous decisions, and also thinking carefully about the future. Remember, all decisions have an element of fantasy and speculation because you must imagine the future. If you will be implementing your decision soon, you probably can anticipate the upcoming circumstances reasonably well. Predicting the distant future, however, is difficult. Even so, there are patterns of events and behaviors that you can use as references to "guesstimate" circumstances that might exist when your decisions will be implemented. Law libraries, business case studies, technical journals, biographies, and government records are a few well-known sources of helpful history. For more personal decisions, you might wish to consult family, friends, and teachers/professors for their knowledge, experience, and input.

The most difficult decisions are those for which no precedent exists or can be found. Other difficult decisions are those that must be made quickly, with little background information. As much as possible, thoughtful processes should accompany all decisions, whether ordinary or extraordinary. Your choices give you a chance to arrange your future according to your desires. With each decision, something else occurs. What you choose to do becomes an expression of who you are—giving you a defining character imprint that you will share with family, friends, and colleagues.

Implementing Your Decision

However, just making a decision is as useless as having an uncracked nut. You have to open it to the world by implementing your decision. Set up an action agenda—what must be done by whom, when, where, why, with what, and how. If you do this right away, you will have better command of your purposes and needs, and the problem is least likely to change before you have a chance to solve it. Flow charts and tree diagrams can be useful. Make sure to include an evaluation or a signal of success into your action agenda so you will know whether you have chosen wisely.

Also, periodically review your decision. A good modern example is the existence of "Sunset Laws" 📖. Governing bodies such as legislatures or committees often set a specific time when they will review a decision that they have made to decide whether or not they want to stay with their decision. Few decisions are irreversible; in almost all situations, change is possible. There are two cautions. The first is to avoid foolish vacillation. Once you make a decision, live with it at least long enough to allow time to prove its worth or worthlessness. The second is to treat yourself kindly. If you decided honestly based on available information, then your decision was the right one—even if it turned out badly. If the results were fantastic, allow yourself a small helping of BLT (the celebrity sandwich known as Bright Lights and Trumpets) and go on as before. Then, get ready for your next decision-making challenge.

Summary

- ▣ Your background—including your personality, knowledge base, cultural and personal experiences, values, and interests—affect your decision-making processes.

- ▣ Problems often have more than one right answer.

- ▣ Avoiding making a decision is itself a decision and can result in an unfavorable outcome.

- ▣ Good decisions can be reached by following one or more procedures.

- ▣ A listing of pros and cons can be a quick aid in making choices.

- ▣ An in-depth process of decision making involves a five-stage method.

- ▣ Decisions need to be followed by action, usually promptly.

- ▣ Periodically review and evaluate your decisions.

Words of Wisdom

The strongest principle of growth lies in human choice.
— George Eliot

Decision is a risk rooted in the courage of being free.
— Paul Tillich

Don't fight the problem; decide it.
— General George C. Marshall

It is a common experience that a problem difficult at night is resolved in the morning after the committee of sleep has worked on it.
— John Steinbeck

Decision is a sharp knife that cuts clean and straight. Indecision is a dull one that hacks and tears and leaves ragged edges behind.
— Jan McKeithen

We have freedom of choice, yes, but not freedom from choice.
— Mary Ellen Edwards

I have accepted fear as a part of life—specifically the fear of change. I have gone ahead despite the pounding in the heart that says: turn back.
— Erica Jong

He will not dither. He will decide. He will not agonize; he will act.
— Hubert H. Humphrey

We know what happens to people who stay in the middle of the road. They get run over.
— Aneurin Bevan

We choose our joys and sorrows long before we experience them.

> – Kahlil Gibran

One thing is sure. We have to do something. We have to do the best we know how at the moment.... If it doesn't turn out right, we can modify it as we go along.

> – Franklin D. Roosevelt

The most difficult thing is the decision to act; the rest is merely tenacity. The fears are paper tigers. You can do anything you decide to do. You can act to change and control your life; and the procedure, the process, is its own reward.

> – Robyn Davidson

Every great decision creates ripples—like a huge boulder dropped in a lake. The ripples merge, rebound off the banks in unforeseeable ways. The heavier the decision, the larger the waves, the more uncertain the consequences.

> – Ben Aaronovitch

If you play it safe in life you've decided that you don't want to grow any more.

> – Shirley Mount Hufstedler

A decision is the action an executive must take when he has information so incomplete that the answer does not suggest itself.

> – Arthur W. Radford

The truth is that many people set rules to keep from making decisions.

> – Mike Krzyzewski

Chapter 8

Frustration: Stress, Depression, and Suicide

When we find ourselves in a frustrating situation, we often feel trapped, powerless, self-critical, and angry. The reaction to frustration is physical as well as mental. Many health professionals believe that high stress levels can result in the accumulation of harmful chemicals in the body, which in turn may lead to migraine headaches, heart attacks, high blood pressure, arthritis, and vision problems. Fatigue, exhaustion, and mental or physical breakdowns are possible. Surprisingly, such physical consequences are not the result of intense and stressful activity when it accompanies successful venture. These chemical "scars" form as a result of stress when it leads to failure—either real or imagined.

Does this mean that you should become so emotionally detached from your environment that nothing ever bothers you? No, but you can learn how to minimize stress, handle it, and turn it to your advantage.

Stress is a Double-Edged Sword

There are times when stress is a good thing. When getting ready to give a speech or other performance in front of an audience, stress can actually bring your efforts to a sharp focus and make your performance better than it would have been without a few "nerves." Stress can also alert you to danger and make your reflexes sharper, as, for example, when you are driving in a rainstorm. Stress can be beneficial because it can bring a focus to your abilities to handle problems or alert you to danger.

Stress is harmful, though, when you inwardly gnaw on it without a creative outlet or a constructive attitude. Knowing what to do when you become frustrated and overloaded by stress can improve your chances of living longer with better health.

Perhaps more immediately debilitating than various physical reactions to stress are the emotional consequences of continued frustration. Unless you learn to manage frustration adequately, the resulting unhappiness, anger, and self-hate you may feel can render you incapable of reacting sensibly.

Turning Things Around

As ironic as it sounds, frustration can be turned into a positive. It allows you to focus on areas of unfairness or incompetence. Your dissatisfaction can allow you to see faulty situations as they really are and then become fuel for a motivational fire to undertake meaningful work. Abraham Lincoln 📖, for example, used his depression as an agent of growth that helped him to develop strength of purpose and conviction.

However, some people use undesirable coping mechanisms for dealing with frustrating situations. One is to regress to early childhood and act like a baby. Typical behaviors of these immature adults include temper tantrums, throwing things, being unreasonably silly, avoiding or ignoring the cause or circumstance of the problem, or pretending not to be frustrated.

Here is one example of possible childish reactions to a problem. Consider that you have lost or mislaid expensive tickets to a concert that you and a friend have looked forward to for a long time. You have forgotten that the tickets are where you put them—in a safe place, under a lamp on your desk. In your frustration, you accuse others of losing them, and you scream at the dog who is begging for dinner while you are searching. You have a desperate "toss on the floor" search through your clothing, and you delay calling your friend until it's too late and she shows up at the door. Then, to cover yourself, you invent a wild story.

In a perfect world, this situation wouldn't happen. Why? Because you would quickly find the tickets, or—even better—you would have such orderly habits that you would always know where your tickets are kept. But this is not a perfect world. It is helpful to remember that there is almost always more than one solution to any problem. Keeping this in mind can help relieve many otherwise stressful situations. When you don't find the tickets, you call your friend, and you rearrange the evening to do something else—a bit less enjoyable, perhaps, but acceptable to both of you.

Another situation involving frustration is one that occurs when moving to a new town. Imagine that you have just moved. In your old town, you were well known and had many friends, but now you know no one. To make the example even more forceful, imagine that you are in a wheelchair. Although in your previous town you had learned ways to easily get around by yourself, now the stairs and narrow doorways in most of the buildings are daily sources of stress. Most frustrating of all, however, is the loneliness. Yet when old friends call, you make believe life is beautiful. In fact, though, you are really avoiding places and people and only pretending that you have an active social life.

Then you discover that e-mail correspondence can be a daily source of joy, and in fact, you organize a chat room. Your difficulty in traveling to inhospitable places now seems less of a frustration. You have found a substitute and reduced the frustration and depression—at least temporarily. Having nearby friends and freedom of movement are still important, but you have found a way to cope with the situation and accept what is, at present, possible. Doing this requires a positive attitude and simplification of desires on your part—both requiring self-discipline and positive ways to deal with stress and frustration.

Sources of Frustration

A catalog of the likely sources of frustration would encompass every known experience—problems with material goods, processes, events, and human relationships. Every change—even a vacation—involves coping, and thus stress. Although the list of possible frustrations is incredibly large, your personal attitude and approach to situations will determine whether or not problems will annoy or baffle you. And remember, someone else may consider the same situations to be challenging, humorous, or unimportant.

Losing, forgetting, or breaking things are common troublesome experiences and are frustrating. Like having accidents, these things may occur more frequently if you are mentally preoccupied. Chronic problems with any of these may be a symptom of other difficulties, and you should try to figure out why they occur (professional help may be advisable). To avoid memory problems, you may find it helpful to make lists of important information.

Ironically, your most stressful experiences may actually be related to your strengths, particularly your creative interests and abilities. Stress might come from:

- Lack of opportunity to use your ability or talent.

- Insufficient access to an education appropriate to your talents and abilities.

- Rejection of your ideas by experts in your field or by a respected teacher.

- Insufficient opportunities to share your abilities with peers or in public settings.

- Personal fear of failure and/or public rejection of your ideas.

- Misappropriation by others of your ideas or creative works.

- Family, social, or cultural constraints ("You can't become a singer because we are a family of lawyers, judges, etc.") or financial constraints ("There isn't enough money.").

- Prejudice of any kind that limits your activity.

- Inability to find someone to help.

- Lack of materials, instruments, or working space.

- Tackling a project too large for your present circumstances.

- Failure of health—physical or mental.

- Having so many interests that focus on any one of them is difficult.

- Failing badly in one endeavor and being unable to decide on a future direction. (Remember, failure is just the discovery of what doesn't work. What will work still exists and is possible.)

- Dealing socially with people who think you are weird because of your creativity or beliefs.

- Criticism by others who feel that you have neglected them.

Stress can come from other good things, too. Even when you are excited about an upcoming event and looking forward to it eagerly, it can still be stressful. For example, weddings, births, getting accepted into the college of your choice, moving into a nicer neighborhood—all of these carry a certain amount of stress with them simply because they signify life-altering changes. Don't berate yourself for feeling stress at significant happy occasions. Allow yourself to have conflicting feelings, and understand that this is natural and expected.

Coping with Frustration

All of these frustrations may seem overwhelming, but they needn't be. The following table lists some possible frustrating attitudes and their "antidotes." Can you relate these suggestions to any of your previous experiences? Would looking at problems in this way have been helpful? You might like to record some of your reactions in your personal notebook.

Attitudes that Often Lead to Frustration	Attitudes that Tend to Decrease Frustration
I can't do anything about this. I'm blocked because:	I can handle this because:
1. I'm powerless.	1. I can find an alternative, obtain help, be patient, or look forward to a day when I will have power. I can learn about how people use or misuse power.
2. No one understands me. No one cares about me.	2. I appreciate being alive—and being able to survive to this point. I am worth a lot just for surviving. I do not expect myself to be perfect or master of every situation. What counts is that I care about myself. There are things that I can do for myself. I'm going to try to be the best there is at x (where x is anything I undertake), because it could be a worthwhile experience.
3. This routine is killing me. It's dull and boring. Sometimes there is too much pressure.	3. I have not made a lifetime commitment to this. I can add something or do something else that gives me some satisfaction or a sense of achievement, even if I have to keep this routine for now.
4. I can't seem to get anything right. I seem to mess up every time.	4. I have confidence in myself. I'll do my best, then let it go if it's impossible. In any case, I'll know more about myself and be more able in the future. My happiness does not depend on someone else's opinion of me, so I don't have to worry about failure. I can ask someone for advice, feedback, or evaluation.

Attitudes that Often Lead to Frustration	Attitudes that Tend to Decrease Frustration
I can't do anything about this. I'm blocked because:	I can handle this because:
5. I wish I could do this, but I don't know how.	5. I can proceed carefully. I've got a chance to do something unusual. Maybe it is risky, and I may not know enough now, but it is a good opportunity to learn and contribute.
6. I can't get what I need or want.	6. Is it really that important? Is there an alternative? Do I really need or want it? Do I have to have it now? Maybe if I am patient, something better will turn up.
7. I can't decide.	7. I would rather make the choice than have someone make it for me. I can find whatever advice or information I need, list the pros and cons, take my time, look at alternatives, and think it through. Whatever decision I make will be the best one possible under these circumstances.
8. I'm too shy or x (x equals anything else I use as an excuse).	8. This is important to me, and I am going to do it. I know it will be tough, but I can try. I'll take one step at a time. If all else fails, I'll try to get someone else to help.
9. No one has ever been in this situation before.	9. Even though this is a unique problem, I know I can find some way to handle it. Maybe this is a good time to brainstorm possible solutions. I can also get some peaceful rest, perhaps observe nature, then approach this problem again. If I need help, I can get it.
10. It is too late. It is hopeless.	10. Even if it is too late this time, I will be better prepared next time. What else can I do? I can do something constructive with what time I have. I can try to make amends for any results of my inaction, perhaps by doing something on a smaller scale.

Suicide

In extreme situations, when everything seems to be going against you and you feel that your situation is hopeless, you may find yourself contemplating suicide. You are not "crazy" if you have ever had suicidal thoughts. Many people have had such thoughts but wisely have not acted upon them. Thinking about suicide can be a reaction to what seems at the time to be an impossible situation, or it can be an angry reaction to a frustrating situation. You may need to realize that virtually all problems are of short duration (at least in their real effect upon you) as long as you are alive. Therefore, thinking about ending your life could be a normal passing thought when you are in a tough situation. But acting upon this impulse is not normal and certainly not desirable. If you have gone so far as to think how you would "do it," you should get help. Help is as near as your phone. Many communities have people who are available to answer telephone calls on a 24-hour basis to provide appropriate counseling. Check the front of your telephone book for this number—usually listed as *Crisis and Suicide Counseling*. The people at these crisis lines have been specially trained to handle calls like this.

Otherwise, talk to someone you trust. Be honest and listen carefully. Suicide has long-lasting and far reaching implications for many different people who have been associated with you. It leaves a wound that never heals for the survivors; this wound is more painful than that left by accidental death or death from an illness. Years later, people may still be hurt because of your choice. Your brothers or sisters may resent that you didn't stick around so that their children could know you. Parents will grieve that you left the world before you discovered your true gift or passion. And while some suicides are done to hurt or "get back at" someone else, as in "I'll show them," the person most hurt of course is the one who kills him- or herself.

As an alternative to this irrevocable act that will affect so many lives besides your own, think of ways to use your considerable talents to help others have a better life. Even if you feel that you have no control over a particular situation, you can learn to manage your viewpoint or attitude about that situation, or you can make a plan to get out of the situation eventually.

One young woman believed that her life was meaningless after her fiancé suffered a suddenly fatal heart attack from an undiagnosed heart condition. She felt that she could never love again, and life without love would be empty. However, a few years later, while working with her community's Healthy Heart Center, she met a sensitive, intelligent man, and she couldn't help but fall in love with him. Had she ended her life, her achievements in the medical field would never have been accomplished, her children would never have been born, and her new-found happiness would never have touched all of the people that she surrounded herself with in her life.

Summary

- ▣ Almost anything can be frustrating.

- ▣ Frustration can affect your mental and physical health.

- ▣ Some stress can be a good thing.

- ▣ Your attitude and knowledge of useful techniques can help you manage troublesome situations.

- ▣ Suicide is never the answer.

- ▣ By being true to yourself and your capacity for contribution, you can convert possible frustrations into opportunities.

Words of Wisdom

Suicide is a permanent solution to a temporary problem.
— Phil Donahue

Man should not try to avoid stress any more than he would shun food, love, or exercise.
— Dr. Hans Selye

The greater part of our happiness or misery depends on our disposition and not on our circumstances.
— Martha Washington

You may be disappointed if you fail, but you are doomed if you don't try.
— Beverly Sills

Post-mortems on defeats are never very useful unless they say something about the future.
— James Reston

When I am hassled about something, I always stop and ask myself what difference it will make in the evolution of the human species in the next ten million years, and that question always helps me to get back my perspective.
— Anne Wilson Schaef

We have to learn to be our own best friends because we fall too easily into the trap of being our own worst enemies.
— Roderick Thorp

Being defeated is often a temporary condition. Giving up is what makes it permanent.
— Marilyn vos Savant

One never notices what has been done; one can only see what remains to be done.
— Marie Curie

What I must do is all that concerns me, not what the people think.
— Ralph Waldo Emerson

Our frustration is greater when we have much and want more than when we have nothing and want some. We are less dissatisfied when we lack many things than when we seem to lack but one thing.
— Eric Hoffer

People need trouble—a little frustration to sharpen the spirit on, toughen it. Artists do; I don't mean you need to live in a rat hole or gutter, but you have to learn fortitude, endurance. Only vegetables are happy.
— William Faulkner.

All blame is a waste of time. No matter how much fault you find with another, and regardless of how much you blame him, it will not change you. The only thing blame does is to keep the focus off you when you are looking for external reasons to explain your unhappiness or frustration. You may succeed in making another feel guilty about something by blaming him, but you won't succeed in changing whatever it is about you that is making you unhappy.
— Wayne Dyer

I've come to believe that all my past failure and frustration were actually laying the foundation for the understandings that have created the new level of living I now enjoy.
— Tony Robbins

Being frustrated is disagreeable, but the real disasters in life begin when you get what you want.
— Irving Kristol

Chapter 9

Brevity and Levity: The Long and the Short of Playing with Words Creatively

Playing with words is a honing process for creative thinking. The main purpose of this chapter is for you to have fun while briefly exploring word games that promote mental flexibility. This pleasant diversion of creativity—the levity of "fooling around"—sometimes results in a worthwhile new idea. But it will be worthwhile even if the only result is your inner sense of satisfaction and enjoyment, perhaps just enjoying the wordplay or perhaps in having solved a puzzle of no great consequence. Many highly creative people have an excellent internal "laugh button" which they use to generate imaginative associations, as well as to maintain a sense of perspective about their world. These people also cultivate opportunities to use their sense of humor when playing games.

The passage quoted below, *Two Unusual Words*, is based on a recording of an actual mental ramble through stored ideas and impressions. It is an illustration of the linking of ideas to one another based on personal knowledge and experience. Everything in this collection of words had personal meaning to the author—and possibly not much significance (as a whole) to anyone else. But to create connections from one phrase to another will require you to flexibly use analytical thought and knowledge, and you may find this to be an interesting challenge. If you find this passage interesting and challenging, you may also enjoy *Mrs. Dalloway* 📖, by Virginia Woolf, which is similar in nature but is a literary classic.

Read *Two Unusual Words* initially without making any serious effort at comprehension. Then continue on and examine *The Cascade Word Game*, and afterward, you might try a few of your own idea sequences. Later, you might come back and enjoy a rereading of *Two Unusual Words*.

Two Unusual Words

*Brevity and levity are unusual words that have similar shapes, sounds, and sizes. Is there a verbal connection, a meaning shared? "Brevity is the soul of **wit**." What is wit? A **wit** is an imaginatively perceptive and articulate individual especially skilled in banter or **persiflage**. **Persiflage**, with a Latin origin meaning hiss, corresponds to **frivolous** or lightly derisive talk or manner of treating a subject. Excessive or unseemly **frivolity** corresponds to **levity**. **Levity** also is the opposite of **gravity**, where **gravity** carries the sense of being weighty or **ponderous**. Then **ponderous** has as synonyms bulky, massive, **huge**, unwieldy, and cumbersome. **Huge** has **small** as an antonym. **Small** can be a synonym for **short**. One of the synonyms for **brevity** is **shortness**. There is a connection! If you think that this hiss has the sibilant sound of a goose, you are mistaken. It is not a wild goose chase even though **sibilare** is Latin for **hiss**.*

*Another turn to take begins with brevity. Digging to the heart of a problem. The briefest way of describing. The least time possible on mundane chores equals an explosion of fun time. Time to **organize** a mental thought flow by linking ideas tersely to produce a valuable entity. Weeks spent producing a ten-word advertising slogan; minutes to write a one-page letter. Personal shorthand. Pruned fruit trees. Satire has a Latin origin (**satura**) meaning a dish filled with various fruit. The ordering of pamplemousse in a Parisian restaurant. (It is not a better variety of chocolate mousse.) Fruit trees—pleached. Word linkage—a mental web. Geese. Feet. The nature of thought processes. Less is more. More is not enough. Sir Thomas More. Becket. T. S. Eliot. **The Wasteland**.*

Time for something else. Levity. Levitation. A balloon ride over the French countryside. Balloon vine. Cardiospermum halicacabum. A sapindaceous tropical climbing plant.

Cardio? Heart. Balloon? Halicacabum! Bum! Sapindaceous. Sap! Light humor. What is ridiculous? Why? Why is laughter contagious? Is laughter essential? Why? Passage from wit to levity. A balloon ride—up, over, and down. The English downs. Sheep. **All Things Bright and Beautiful.** *Beautiful laughter. Laughter in the place of anger. Laughter to preserve sanity. A cleanser. Abrasive. Polish. A polished speech. The introductory joke.* **The Modern Handbook of Humor.** *Dr. George Harris, addressing an assembly at Amherst College: "I intended to give you some advice, but now I remember how much is left over from last year unused." The place of honor in a procession is at the end. Rosebuds. Robert Herrick. The quest ends demonstrative. Stop.*

The playfulness inherent in the idea sequence of *Two Unusual Words* can be achieved almost anywhere, anytime. No equipment is needed except you—no game board, no racquet, no special shoes. A mind teeming with ideas, memories, recallable sights, facts, and words, is all that is necessary. Playing this mental game involves a cascade of your thoughts, starting either with a word that is of personal interest or a word selected randomly—perhaps from a book, selection of photographs, fabric swatch book, tool catalog, seed list, etc.

Cascade Word Game

Consider the following word sequences as examples of the *Cascade Word Game*. They are brief digressions involving word associations. They start with the first word and, by simple association, come to the word below it and so forth until the process reaches a creative end. The search for the next word involves you thinking of, and then discarding, ideas that are not personally suitable until something finally "clicks" and you find a word you like.

This mind-stretching game can be played easily in brief moments of solitude. Unlike the nearly constant and often rambling internal mental chatter going on in our minds, this thinking is more organized and deliberate. With this, like all games, some results are better than others. Try aiming at occasional silliness and verbal slapstick. Like jazz, it is disciplined and yet creative. Explore the *Cascade Word Game* often, perhaps as a way to make standing in line somewhere more interesting. Record some of your best efforts in your personal notebook.

Example 1

Brevity
Brief
Leif
Lief
Laugh
Cry

In this first example, a near synonym of *brevity* begins the cascade with the word *brief.* The ending sound brief, brought *Leif* to mind (Leif Ericson, Viking explorer 📖), and this was bounced to *lief* (which means gladly, willingly), which led to *laugh*, and then its sensory antonym, *cry*.

Example 2

Levity
Lever
Ever
Ere
Verity
Very

In this second example, a quick response to *levity* was *lever* because of the similar verbal beginning. Then the word *ever* was an easy choice since it was enclosed in *lever*. A bit of mental maneuvering produced *ere* (meaning before). Then the easy process ended. *Ere* produced no immediate response. A mental shuffling of shapes, sounds, and meanings occurred with a scanning of all of the preceding words. *Verity* (meaning truth) popped up next. Searching backwards, *ever* yielded *ver.* A visual alignment with the shape and size of *levity* led to *verity*. Quickly, *very* formed as a final word out of both ends of *verity*.

The *Cascade Word Game* is a playful but disciplined way to explore relationships within your personal knowledge bank. Although these two examples of word cascades were developed using the key chapter words, *brevity* and *levity*, any other set of words or terms could have been used. The purpose of making these mental chains is to trigger mental searching processes; partly conscious, partly unconscious; partly emotional, partly analytical.

Finally, the terms *brevity* and *levity* may encourage you to think about the nature of discovery. Kary Mullis 📖, a Nobel Laureate in chemistry, refers to this process of investigation as follows: "Simplicity is embarrassing when you have to work for months to achieve it. You…will wonder why people get the Nobel Prize for pointing out such simple things. The answer is that most people can't see the simple things and the simple things are always the most important." Perhaps the *Cascade Word Game* will help you in discovering the important simple things in your life and how to do so with levity.

Summary

- The briefest and best possible statement often requires the most intense examination of many ideas.

- Your ability to create order depends upon the amount of disorder that you can comfort- ably store and eventually rearrange.

- Accumulate ideas like a pack rat; try using ideas in the Cascade Word Game instead of single words.

- Use levity as a pry bar to stir up your mental collection of data.

Words of Wisdom

As long as one keeps searching, the answers come.
— Joan Baez

[It was] an initiation into the love of learning, of learning how to learn, that was revealed to me by my BLS masters as a matter of interdisciplinary cognition—that is, learning to know something by the relation to something else.
— Leonard Bernstein

Life forms illogical patterns. It is haphazard and full of beauties which I try to catch as they fly by, for who knows whether any of them will ever return?
— Margot Fonteyn

The clouds gathered together, stood still and watched the river scuttle around the forest floor, crash headlong into haunches of hills with no notion of where it was going, until exhausted, ill and grieving, it slowed to a stop just twenty leagues short of the sea.
— Toni Morrison

When I am playful, I use the meridians of longitude and parallels of latitude for a seine, and drag the Atlantic Ocean for whales. I scratch my head with the lightning and purr myself to sleep with the thunder.
— Mark Twain

No day in which you learn something is a complete loss.
— David Eddings

I never learn anything talking. I only learn when I ask questions.
— Lou Holtz

The test of a first-rate intelligence is the ability to hold two opposed ideas in the mind at the same time, and still retain the ability to function.
— F. Scott Fitzgerald

Piling up knowledge is as bad as piling up money. You have to begin sometime to kick around what you know.
— Robert Frost

My method is to take the utmost trouble to find the right thing to say, and then to say it with the utmost levity.
— Georg Bernard Shaw

In my experience sometimes the darker the material that you're doing, the more necessary it is to have some sort of levity around.
— Nick Stahl

Be sincere; be brief; be seated.
— Franklin D. Roosevelt

The most valuable of all talents is that of never using two words when one will do.
— Thomas Jefferson

Wise men talk because they have something to say; fools talk because they have to say something.
— Plato

Words are, of course, the most powerful drug used by mankind.
— Rudyard Kipling

Chapter 10

Self-Esteem: Mastering Your Own Challenges

Although self-esteem fluctuates, you are never without it. It is your psychological barometer, responding to the pressures of daily life much as your outer skin responds to physical pressure. Just as a healthy outer skin is a desirable entity, so too is a healthy inner self-esteem. With it, even miserable days can be valuable.

On some days, you find both shoes, walk out into a beautiful sunny morning, say exactly the right things to someone, and hear exactly what you wish to hear in return. You smile going to sleep. On other days, the shoes still fit, but nothing else does. Your reactions to the good and the bad, the expected and unexpected, your moods and the moods of others—all of these contribute to your "inner self" and your self-esteem.

So how do you develop a healthy self-esteem? You accept the fact that truly doing your best each day provides the real definition of your success. Your best may not correspond to someone else's standard of perfection, but it doesn't have to. Remember that perfectionism is by definition illogical. Omniscience and infallibility are not attainable human characteristics.

However, truly doing your best each day in matters that are important can be a real challenge that requires honesty and effort. Honesty dictates that you make efforts consistent with everything that you know about yourself and your surroundings. Effort involves striving for effectiveness in your immediate daily activities, as well as a consciously planned preparation for the future. Preparation for the future implies not only a projected image of yourself in that future, but also an awareness of what might be required for you to arrive at that future state.

The preceding sentence describes an enormous complexity—sufficient to occupy your attention for the rest of your life. One complication is that you must know yourself. Events in childhood, and afterward, help shape your perception of yourself. That perception can be warped. For example, if you were an overprotected child and kept from situations in which you would have to make decisions, you may not currently respect your own judgment capabilities. That doesn't mean that you cannot choose wisely; it only means that you may have to develop this skill by trial and error now, since you did not have opportunities to do so earlier.

If you grew up in a constantly critical atmosphere, you may believe that anything less than perfection is just not good enough. Since you have accepted external, perfectionistic standards that are unrealistic, you may try to do very little, knowing that you can never "measure up." As a result, you may feel worthless. However, by making a determined effort to refute this burden of perfectionism, you *can* function very capably. Although a message such as "Needs better organization" on a paper or report may convey a lack of worth to you, it may not have been intended that way. Some comments, which you might take very personally, may have been intended simply as helpful constructive criticism.

When you hear yourself thinking: "I'm always wrong," "I failed; what's the use in trying," "If only I'd had the sense to…"; STOP. Tell yourself instead: "I've been right many times before. This mistake teaches me that there is a different answer from the one I chose. I'll remember the right answer for this occasion. This mistake doesn't erase all of my previous successes, nor does it foretell future failures. I've just got some more learning to do."

You need to realize your own worthiness—that you are a good person with a unique set of talents and abilities. *Everyone* is special, *everyone* can enjoy each day, and *everyone* can add something to the total sum of human experience. You must absorb this idea deeply into yourself—your "inner skin" has to accept the impression that you are okay. And remember that feeling okay has to be cultivated.

Elements of Self-Esteem

Self-esteem is a combination of self-confidence and self-respect. Self-confidence develops from repeated successful experiences in handling events, in interacting with people, and in making good daily choices. Self-respect depends on being honorable in your daily actions, in accord with principles or standards that you have accepted and developed for your personal use. In fact, William James 📖, the father of modern psychology, developed a formula for self-esteem more than 100 years ago:

$$Self\text{-}Esteem = Success/Pretensions$$

That is, we can feel better about ourselves either by succeeding more in the world or by lowering our expectations and hopes (i.e., our pretensions). Of course, reducing your self-expectations seldom develops realistic self-esteem; we rarely feel good when we accomplish something that we already can easily do. Instead, self-esteem comes from mastering a task that has some challenge.

Consider, as an example, the choices made by a very successful musician who "reworked" material developed by lesser-known contemporaries. The recognition that he receives contributes to his self-confidence in stage appearances. He may believe that his creativity is honorable—that he has a legitimate reason to build upon the ideas of others. In this case, his self-respect and his self-esteem may be high. But suppose he knows that his success is dishonorable, based on his fraudulent efforts to claim undeserved originality. If this bothers him, his self-respect and self-esteem will suffer despite his success. Although there are some universal standards of behavior, it is the individual's awareness and acceptance of these standards that determine his regard for himself.

Now consider a not-so-successful musician. If he has faith in his ability, he continues to write music, has high self-esteem, and confidently continues to work hard despite limited recognition. But if he knowingly makes minimal efforts to produce original compositions, his sense of self-worth diminishes, and he may need to re-examine his choice of occupation.

The way in which these two musicians react to criticism probably varies. As self-esteem plunges, over-reaction and defensive responses to criticism tend to rise. In contrast, a confident person can see criticism as a potentially useful information source.

Some situations will require you to give extra attention and care to issues of self-esteem. You might be an innovator, an explorer, or someone working at the interface of the new and the old. Other people may view your wonderful discoveries as bizarre, unimportant, and useless. But if you believe in your efforts and their value, your self-esteem is less likely to crumple.

If you can do many things with better-than-average ease, you may attempt more than is practical, and you may end up overworked or feeling used. Other people may take advantage of your abilities by offering you many special tasks that will take "only a few minutes." Learn how to be selective so that you can do justice to whatever you undertake. If you tackle too much and just achieve mediocrity, your self-esteem may suffer.

When you excel at something, take care that you do not become so absorbed that you forget to respond to the efforts of others or recognize the contributions of others in that area. It is possible to focus on a task so exclusively that you become nearly totally self-contained and unresponsive to outside influences. This self-absorption may simply come from a fascination with the projects at hand. But sometimes a focus on achievements can actually be a form of trophy-hunting and a need for approval—a symptom of low self-esteem.

All of us experience times when we feel disappointed in our efforts or when our efforts are not valued or appreciated by others. Sometimes we may even be strongly criticized. This can cause us to change our self-perceived status from high to low. What happens then to your level of self-esteem? *It need not and should not decrease.* Although we should be open to evaluation from others or from within ourselves, this doesn't need to drastically influence our self-esteem. Self-esteem is self-described and self-contained. You are yourself—you do not increase or decrease in ability because of the opinions of others. You should listen to these opinions but validate yourself based on an inner integrity. Value the importance of achieving rather than the competitiveness that may lead to achievement.

Finally, you may fear that if you depend on others, it is an indication of weakness or low self-esteem. But remember, no one is omniscient, infallible, or completely self-reliant. By sharing abilities, insights, and efforts, the sum becomes greater than its parts. You have much to offer. Others do also.

Maintaining and Improving Self-Esteem

The following is a list of some of the things that you can do to maintain and improve your self-esteem. Try any that interest you.

- Keep a scrapbook, picture album, or personal notebook to record achievement and point toward future possibilities.

- Develop a hobby or recreational interest that you can turn to when other occupations become troublesome.

- Practice giving deserved compliments to others. As you perceive the good in others, so too will you be more sensitive to your own goodness.

- Regard failures as learning experiences. You will learn what you *can* do—not just what you cannot do.

- If all things that you do are easy, then you need to move to areas that are *not* so easy. Unless you stretch yourself, how else will you really find out what you can do?

- Plan to enjoy something each day. Respond to something pleasurable to revive your spirit.

- Make an inventory of your assets. Look at them occasionally. What can you do very well? What have you accomplished?

- Work at self-improvement. Consider what you can do to overcome handicaps or compensate for weaknesses. Set goals, and develop a plan of action. Decide to do something by a certain date; put it on your personal calendar.

- Associate with optimistic people.

- Read literature, including time-proven works of art that can extend your awareness of "the human condition."

- Picture yourself as being what you want to be—what you believe is the real you. Do this as a mental exercise before undertaking any serious task.

◼ Surround yourself with positive suggestions. Plant sayings, proverbs, catch phrases, or personal exhortations in your purse or wallet, on a notebook, in your desk, on a mirror frame, or wherever you are likely to find them easily.

◼ Regularly plan to give something, while expecting nothing in return. Giving will help you realize the vitality of your inner core and your accomplishments.

◼ Recognize that being assertive is a non-aggressive act. It is a compassionate revelation of self—a willingness to extend outward to accept and share responsibilities. Join a group or association that will permit your active, assertive participation.

◼ Set up rewards for yourself. Do something special to celebrate accomplishments.

◼ Create a private salvage system for your days of low self-esteem. It may include talking to someone for reassurance, reading something humorous or inspirational, or spending time doing something that you really like to do and do well. Have this system established in advance of need, and make sure that it really adds to your well-being.

Summary

◼ The desire for self-esteem is basic to life.

◼ A healthy self-esteem develops when you do your best each day.

◼ Your perception of reality affects how you regard yourself.

◼ Self-esteem comes as you master challenges

◼ You need to recognize and address problems that may arise because of your talented nature.

◼ Certain activities will enhance your acceptance of yourself.

Words of Wisdom

Don't compromise yourself. You are all you've got.
— Janis Joplin

I desire so to conduct the affairs of this administration that if at the end, when I come to lay down the reins of power, I have lost every other friend on earth, I shall at least have one friend left, and that friend shall be down inside of me.
— Abraham Lincoln

When we can begin to take our failures nonseriously, it means we are ceasing to be afraid of them. It is of immense importance to learn to laugh at ourselves.
— Katherine Mansfield

Nobody can make you feel inferior without your consent.
— Eleanor Roosevelt

Be yourself. No one can ever tell you're doing it wrong.
— James Leo Herlihly

Every time we start thinking we're the center of the universe, the universe turns around and says with a slightly distracted air, "I'm sorry. What'd you say your name was again?"
— Margaret Maron

Love yourself first and everything else falls into line. You really have to love yourself to get anything done in this world.
— Lucille Ball

Always be a first-rate version of yourself, instead of a second-rate version of somebody else.
— Judy Garland

Ninety percent of the world's woe comes from people not knowing themselves, their abilities, their frailties, and even their real virtues. Most of us go almost all the way through life as complete strangers to ourselves—so how can we know anyone else?

– Sydney J. Harris

Your chances of success in any undertaking can always be measured by your belief in yourself.

– Robert Collier

Nothing builds self-esteem and self-confidence like accomplishment.

– Thomas Carlyle

Self-esteem isn't everything; it's just that there's nothing without it.

– Gloria Steinem

Just as we develop our physical muscles through overcoming opposition—such as lifting weights—we develop our character muscles by overcoming challenges and adversity.

– Stephen R. Covey

You'll never know your limits until you try to extend them, and even then, one has to break out of his/her comfort zone to appreciate that effort.

– Martin Dansky

Simply put, you believe that things and people make you unhappy, but this is not accurate. You make yourself unhappy.

– Wayne Dyer

There are some people who live in a dream world, and there are some who face reality; and then there are those who turn one into the other.

– Douglas H. Everett

Chapter 11

Conversational Skills: More than Just Listening and Speaking

Do you realize that those who succeed, who are promoted to important positions, or who are popular at social gatherings are often those who talk engagingly and distinctively? Others of equal potential are sometimes overlooked, not because they lack interesting ideas, but because they lack conversational skills.

There are three aims of conversation: (1) simply to enjoy interacting with other people, (2) to get to know the other person better, including how he or she thinks and feels, and (3) to build trust and credibility to develop friendships and relationships.

As with any skill, practice is needed in the art of smooth and interesting conversation. Additionally, it is important to recognize that mental stability, perspective, and self-understanding often derive from daily contact with people; thus, all human interactions are valuable. Even if you are very busy, include some social occasions in your schedule. Take advantage of conversational opportunities.

Here are some guidelines that may help you become a better conversationalist:

- Maintain appropriate body language, including looking at people and maintaining a reasonable amount of eye contact.

- Avoid all self-enclosing gestures, such as folded arms or hiding behind a book, and noise-making movements such as chewing gum.

- Have a friendly face that is alert, obviously receptive, and smiling when appropriate.

◙ Stand before a mirror and practice smiling with your mouth closed. Your eye openings and facial appearance change; you *look* pleasant. When you look at someone that way, they will want to talk with you.

◙ Address the person you are talking to by name. People seldom get tired of hearing their name, and they react warmly.

◙ At the end of the conversation, thank the other person. Closing statements like, "I enjoyed talking with you," "Thanks for letting me know," or, "I appreciated hearing your thoughts" encourage a person to want to talk to you again.

Of course, you don't want to talk all the time. Listening is a key part of any good conversation. And when you do talk, you don't want to be a bore. What good is all of your rich, internalized wisdom and knowledge if you often say trite, tiresome, or depressing things? Make use of the following guidelines on every possible occasion. As in most activities, thoughtful practice and self-awareness will help you succeed.

Don't Chatter or Talk Constantly

Let others have their chance. Find a subject of interest to the *other* person. This will diminish your self-consciousness and will please the other person. It also gives you the best opportunity to learn something; thus, everyone wins.

Don't Be Chronically Silent

The perpetual listener is often thought of as being dull, uninterested, and/or unfriendly. When listening, look at the speaker, occasionally nod your head, or add a brief comment to show interest.

Select a Subject and Intelligently Pursue It

At tonight's dinner table, catch the first thought of general interest and direct it to someone. If you receive no response, ask a question. Try to stay with this topic as long as possible, perhaps 30 minutes. Prolonged examination of a topic changes superficial chitchat into valuable conversation.

Don't chase after a subject that no one else is interested in, however. People will learn to avoid speaking with you if they think that you will trap them in seemingly unending conversations that bore them.

Guide Conversation

Ask yourself: "Will anyone remember this conversation tomorrow?" If not, try to change the subject tactfully to something more useful or relevant. Even tiresome comments on weather can be deflected toward economics, science, art, or almost any other area if you are imaginative. Be prepared to effect such a change. Consider the following exchange:

"It has been a really hot summer."
"Do you think it is exceptional?"
"As far as I am concerned, yes."

Possible directing response:

"Does it make you believe in the Greenhouse Effect 📖 ?"

Another possible technique is to ask advice *sincerely.* This is a great way to redirect a superficial conversation.

X:	*"Omigod! Did you see the outfits those band members were wearing? They were so tacky and ancient!"*
You:	*"Oh, before I forget, I need your advice. Should we set up that meeting with John?"*
X:	*"Well, next Saturday afternoon would be okay. As I was saying."*
You:	*"Do you think that John's idea is sensible? Can we get it done before December?"*

The net result is a conversation guided toward something mutually useful. Yet another way to change the subject or enliven a dying conversation is by using an item of scenery or circumstance to draw the speaker's attention to a new topic.

Introduce Others into the Conversation

When practical, welcome newcomers to a group conversation by mentioning their names. This may help encourage other members of the group (who may not know or remember the names of the new persons) to include them. Then try to help newcomers become aware of the current topic, perhaps by restating a key point from earlier in the conversation, and invite them to join in.

Develop Interesting Ideas

Your personal notebook can be a rich source of conversational gambits. Reserve a section to record unusual facts, notable quotes, book titles, items related to your work, or items of interest to friends. Try to make one abbreviated entry per day for a month. Observe, read, or think of something each day that you consider exciting.

One of the best ways to be prepared with interesting ideas for conversational topics is to read the local newspaper regularly. If time is short, scan headlines and lead paragraphs. Regularly read a few unusual magazines. Become familiar with current bestsellers, and read as many of these books as time and taste allow. Know something about your neighborhood—past or upcoming concerts, art exhibits, sports events, plays, and lectures. Watch television specials.

Psychological research suggests that as much as 80% of all of our conversation is trivial, aimless, and filled with clichés! For instance, remarks about a television program in terms of cast, program length, and time of broadcast are often insignificant. Talking about what the program meant to you or what kinds of questions it raised is more likely to be meaningful. For example, if a friend is interested in architecture, discussing a TV special on Frank Lloyd Wright 📖 could be mutually enjoyable and worthwhile.

With some thought, you can almost immediately discover one or more conversational subjects that interest people. Some helpful conversation openers could range from "What did you do last weekend?" to "If you had an extra hundred dollars to spend tomorrow, what would you do?" Think up some similar openers suitable to your conversation circles.

Younger people generally like to discuss the present and the future; older people often like to discuss the past. Be prepared to give and take at each end of the time spectrum. The rich brocade of the past is best woven by those who lived in it, while the gauzy wings of the future fly wildly in young dreams. Instead of becoming impatient with narratives derived from the "good-old-days," encourage them. You will never have a better chance to learn that kind of history—intensely personalized. The events you read about in books become real when you listen to someone who actually was there. Likewise, when futuristic ideas irritate you because they seem too far-fetched, stir up your own imagination. Try to "top" them, and you will probably end up having some real fun.

Avoid Sensitive Subjects

Try to avoid potentially argumentative subjects unless you are very well acquainted with the other person. Especially in group situations, avoid personal subjects such as weight, personal habits, or appearance that might hurt feelings or lead to gossip sessions. Religious beliefs, politics, or personal relationships may also be controversial and thus difficult subjects to discuss in certain situations.

Develop Vocabulary

Work at building an interesting word supply. Deliberately strike overworked words and terms from your speech, and teach yourself to use substitutes. Some common repetitive terms include "okay," "like," "really," "no way," or "you know."

What you say in casual conversation with friends usually requires a slightly different vocabulary than what you use when you are speaking in more formal occasions, such as an interview. However, in both cases, interesting and appropriate words will mark you as being someone special and worth listening to.

Alexander Hamilton 📖 once gave a speech in New York City that earned him a reputation as an intelligent politician and potential statesman. He was 17 years old! Fifteen years later in 1789, at age 32, he became the first United States Secretary of the Treasury.

Speeches and conversations show a sense of a person's character. Mr. Hamilton's use of language earned him the respect of his listeners. Your determination to learn new words and use them with precision and skill may likewise earn you the respect of your listeners.

Cultivate a Pleasant Voice

It is difficult to concentrate on what someone is saying if you are distracted by how their voice sounds. You may want to check your voice by recording it while reading something interesting. Experiment with changes in pitch and volume. Try to express emotion appropriately. Then listen to yourself. Consult Internet and library sources for remediation if you sound breathy, harsh, whiny, squeaky, or non-melodious. Breathing exercises can help. There are also resources available if you have a speech impediment, which can be extremely distracting to many listeners.

Listen carefully to how public speakers talk. Skilled speakers know how to change volume and pacing to maintain interest. Try doing this. You will be interested to discover how you can influence the pace of a conversation simply by changing your own speech rate and loudness.

Control Diction

When listening to your voice recording, check for enunciation. Can you understand each word? Are contracted words clear? Does "going to" sound like "gonna"? Pay attention to final d's and t's. Others often assess your cultural background by your speech. Sloppy speech may indicate a sloppy mind.

Summary

- ▣ Seek conversational opportunities.

- ▣ Adopt a receptive physical appearance.

- ▣ Be neither the monopolist nor the minimalist.

- ▣ Nurture an interesting subject to make it fruitful.

- ▣ Aim at making the conversation worthwhile.

- ▣ Prepare a richly furnished mind.

- ▣ Select topics wisely.

- ▣ Use the best possible tools: an appropriate vocabulary, a pleasant voice, and precise diction.

Words of Wisdom

Bore: a person who talks when you wish him to listen.
— Ambrose Bierce

The wit of conversation consists much less in showing a great deal of it than in bringing it out in others.
— La Bruyere

Television permits us to walk through life with minor speaking parts. And the more we fail to speak, the more difficult speaking becomes.
— Lois Wyse

Nothing lowers the level of conversation more than raising the voice.
— Stanley Horowitz

The true spirit of conversation consists in building on another man's observation, not overturning it.
— Edward G. Bulwer-Lytton

The real art of conversation is not to say the right thing in the right place, but to leave unsaid the wrong thing at the tempting moment.
— Dorothy Nevill

The value of the average conversation could be enormously improved by the constant use of four simple words: "I do not know."
— Andre Maurois

Conversation means being able to disagree and still continue the discussion.
— Dwight MacDonald

Silence may be as variously shaded as speech.
— Edith Wharton

*Good communication is as stimulating as black coffee—
and just as hard to sleep after.*
— Anne Morrow Lindbergh

Two monologues do not make a dialogue.
— Jeff Daly

*It was impossible to get a conversation going; everybody
was talking too much.*
— Yogi Berra

*A high-school girl, seated next to a famous astronomer at a
dinner party, struck up a conversation with him by asking:
"What do you do for a living?" "I study astronomy," he
replied. "Really?" said the teenager, wide-eyed. "I finished
astronomy last year."*
— James Keller

*Conversation: A vocal competition in which the one who is
catching his breath is called the listener.*
— Ambrose Bierce

Chapter 12

Communication Beyond Words: Body Language and Appearance

You come home late, slam the door, and fail to respond to a pleasant greeting. Or you come home late, have a tense look on your face, sit stiffly, and respond curtly to your family's greeting. These two vignettes are so similar that, if you were acting in a play, it might take a skilled director to know which one of your portrayals interpreted a role more correctly.

You say that you are neither a director nor an actor. But you do present yourself daily to others through your actions and appearance. How? Perhaps on a particular day something wonderful and extraordinary has occurred. But in response to the friendly question, "How are you doing?" you attempt to look nonchalant and hide your excitement, answering, "Oh, I'm okay." Your close friend will know that something is up, however, because your actions are animated and your eyes are bright. Your facial and body language have been more revealing than your words and have given you away.

Appearance and actions are keys in communications between people. In fact, body language, appearance, and tone of voice are the primary ways for communicating emotions. More important than what we say is how we say it and how we look, and our appearance and actions strongly influence how others will react to us. How can you improve your interactions with others? First, develop skill in reading faces and body language. Second, know yourself as you appear and choose to appear to others.

Learn to Read Faces and Body Language

There are many "dictionaries" for body language—books and Internet articles that discuss in depth how what you say with your movements and expressions is often times "louder" than what you say in words. Search out some of the modern references that exist, especially those that are well illustrated. When you visit an art gallery, look for subtleties in the figures and faces of people portrayed by sensitive artists. Critically watching movies and television, possibly with the sound turned off, can increase your awareness of body language and its relationship to verbal language. How close, for example, do the people stand to each other? Where are they looking? How tight are lips? Assess acting that is believable, and observe people on various talk shows. Become more aware of the body movements of people who you meet and what those movements might convey. You might imagine yourself to be a detective of body cues.

Certain appearances are desirable in normal social situations because these patterns have commonly accepted meanings in our culture. For instance, frequently looking directly at someone when talking to them suggests honesty and interest in their reactions. Some body language is complex in its meaning. For example, a smile can sometimes be so brief that it is insincere, or it can be so long that it is a prolonged foolish grin. A sincere smile has a retention span that is just right. Try to observe this in people who are socially adept, and then practice your own smile. The psychologist Paul Ekman 📖 has spent his professional career studying nonverbal communication and found that most facial expressions of emotion are universal, rather than culturally determined. He also found that facial "microexpressions" and other body language can reliably be used to detect lying, and he has used this research to train police officers.

Evaluate Your Own Body Language

Evaluate the length of your walking stride, your posture, and the swinging of your arms. In conversations, notice your hand movements, eye opening, head angles, shrug styles, crossing of legs, manner of sitting, touching of hair or clothing, handling small objects, and folding of arms, plus innumerable combinations of those expressions that convey information about you. When you meet people for the first time, such as on interviews, you are judged initially by your appearance. There is an alert look that accompanies intelligence that is hard to fake, as opposed to a blank stare. A vibrant, lively face, coupled with disciplined body movements, projects a desirable image and is charismatic.

Surprisingly, your face can be shaped by choice—to some extent. By relaxing certain muscles, your lips look fuller and your face appears more "open." The narrowing of eyes or the raising of the forehead, when habitually practiced, produces a certain "set" to the face. Just as your handwriting changes as you mature, so too does your face in response to a maturing personality.

Be careful, however. What is considered good form in one social setting or culture may be offensive in another. In the Near East, people generally stand closer to each other than would be customary in other areas of the world. The private space of an individual is wider in the United States. Standing too close in the U.S. is an affront; standing too far away in the Near East is an insult or a sign of coldness. In some cultures, arm grabbing and hugging are an essential part of any greeting. In other cultures, this is offensive. You will become aware of these differences if you travel or interact within different cultural groups.

Body actions that tend to minimize below-the-neck attention are considered evidence of social grace. Thus, large arm movements, sprawling body positions, and sexually suggestive motions are undesirable. There is logic to this. A sensitive person thinks that taking up more space than necessary is an imposition to be avoided. Also, any actions that increase facial attention will make sure that verbal communication is accurately received. Body language should enhance, even reinforce, the integrity of the spoken word as economically as possible. Repetitive body movements, such as obvious gum chewing, foot tapping, and hand swinging, are particularly irritating gestures to many people. Probably the best advice is to not chew gum at all in public—unless you can do so *very* discreetly.

Some of your distinctive gestures may be the result of unconscious mimicry of family members or friends. Try to be aware of what these mannerisms communicate to others. If they seem to irritate or offend others, practice until you delete them.

Look for Synchrony

When people feel comfortable with each other—or even when they simply *want* to be comfortable with each other—they tend to mimic each other's actions. If one person crosses her legs, the other person will cross hers. If one person leans forward, the other person will lean forward as well. This synchrony occurs even in speech. If one person speaks rapidly or loudly, the other person is likely to speak the same way. The synchrony phenomenon holds for speech rate, loudness, pauses, and length of a person's statement.

Synchrony can be a key piece of information when you are talking to someone. If the synchrony is not there, then some discomfort probably exists between the people involved. Perhaps the other person somehow feels put off by you or believes that you are not a person that he or she wants to know well.

Outward Appearances Speak Loudly

Spiky technicolor hair, partially shaved heads, very long locks, tattoos, and body piercings all have been used as statements to assert independence and convey individualism. At a minimum, a hairdo suggests the extent to which you are interested in yourself and your self-image. Hairstyles can be elaborate, distinctive, time-consuming, simple, contemporary, youthful, and all of the contrary descriptions. Just remember that how you present yourself is essentially how you "advertise" yourself to others, and so your hairstyle—as well as the rest of your appearance, such as makeup (for women) or facial hair (for men)—should be both comfortable and in keeping with your personality and how you want others to see you.

Clothing provides another medium for self-projection. What works for an artist such as Louise Nevelson 📖, Elton John 📖, or Salvador Dali 📖 would be unseemly for a politician or an engineer. Social expectation sets standards and limits for public dress. One of the most scientific dress code explicators is John T. Molloy 📖. His books are widely available and may be of interest to you. What you choose to wear will change with the formality of a situation. Jeans worn for everyday are rarely suitable to be worn at employment interviews.

Make your daily grooming as complete as possible. An unkempt appearance conveys to others that you do not particularly care about yourself or about them. Of course, be clean and use fragrances sparingly. An overpowering perfume or lotion can repel, rather than attract, other people.

Finally, remember that there is a time and a place for everything. Some people who wear suits to the office every day enjoy the freedom of putting on leather jackets and chaps after work for a motorcycle gathering with friends. In both settings, these individuals are dressed acceptably, yet neither style of dress would be appropriate in the alternate setting. Being able to customize your appearance based on what you are doing and who you are doing it with is the essence of creative self-expression with your appearance. Likewise, tattoos may need to be covered and piercings removed in certain social situations, but you should feel free to express yourself (within the boundaries of what is physically healthy) when you are able to do so.

Record in your personal notebook any changes in your appearance that you may want to consider or attempt as a result of reading this chapter.

Summary

- Appearance and actions are key aspects of communication.

- Knowledge of body language can help you communicate more effectively.

- Certain facial expressions and body movements are associated with relatively precise cultural meanings.

- You can consciously modify your total appearance.

- Your appearance may affect your ability to accomplish your goals.

Words of Wisdom

Eat to please thyself, but dress to please others.
— Benjamin Franklin

The outward form the inward man reveal,
We guess the pulp before we cut the peel.
— Oliver Wendell Holmes

They (the English) think him the best dressed man, whose dress is so fit for his use that you cannot notice or remember to describe it.
— Ralph Waldo Emerson

Try to be like the turtle—at ease in your own shell.
— Bill Copeland

Why not be oneself? That is the whole secret of a successful appearance. If one is a greyhound, why try to look like a Pekinese?
— Edith Sitwell

A winning smile is the best accessory any dress ever had.
— C. Terry Cline, Jr.

To live content with small means; to seek elegance rather than luxury, and refinement rather than fashion.
— William Henry Channing

Beautiful faces are those that wear whole-souled honesty printed there.
— Ellen P. Allerton

The weirder you're going to behave, the more normal you should look. It works in reverse, too. When I see a kid with three or four rings in his nose, I know there is absolutely nothing extraordinary about that person.
— P. J. O'Rourke

I agree that a well groomed appearance or a slovenly appearance says a lot about one's character.
— Gloria Gaynor

The most common error made in matters of appearance is the belief that one should disdain the superficial and let the true beauty of one's soul shine through. If there are places on your body where this is a possibility, you are not attractive—you are leaking.
— Charles Lamb

The biggest fool in the world is he who merely does his work supremely well, without attending to appearance.
— Michael Korda

There was a period of time where I tried to cut my hair and dye it and change my appearance, but I realize that in the end, you look better in a specific way and people are always going to pass judgment on you, so it's really up to them to see you in the light that you want to be seen.
— Kristanna Loken

Chapter 13

Organizing Meetings: Like Herding Cats

Chance encounters sometimes profoundly affect humanity. One such encounter took place between two scientists on a commuter train in Germany in the early 1900s, and this encounter eventually led to the development of the Quantum Theory of Atomic Structure 📖. In turn came the search for new elements, the study of nuclear processes, the atomic bomb, and atomic energy plants. Not all meetings are as casual or as fruitful. However, meetings can be interesting and useful if executed properly.

As an instigator of ideas, a trailblazer, an entrepreneur, you will need to know how to organize meetings. Why? Shared ideas are more influential. Sharing hones ideas, sharpening, correcting, and modifying them. Those ideas that survive public scrutiny tend to inspire activity. In our complex society, lobbies and groups of people best effect change—even though the original spark usually comes from one person. Consider the history of environmental concern and the contributions of Rachel Carson 📖 and of Lois Gibbs 📖. Carson's book, *Silent Spring*, took a long time to have an effect on public attitudes about the environment. Gibbs took the route of holding public meetings on Love Canal 📖 and had more immediate results with respect to environmental change. Of course, the influence of Rachel Carson's work probably made people more responsive to the efforts of Lois Gibbs. Therefore, the difference in their methods was not the only factor affecting the results.

You, too, may have passionate beliefs that you would like to share in a public forum. Have you considered the possibility of organizing a meeting with you as a speaker? You might enlist others to present similar or opposing views. You might be able to arrange a public debate with the help of someone serving as moderator. Ideas come from people and then become agents of change when they are publicly shared. If you really want to bring about change, consider meetings as a means of doing this. Even very small audiences can provide a useful forum for your ideas. Begin by discussing your ideas with your family and close friends. Seek their advice concerning sharing your ideas with other people.

Sometimes, the need to hold a meeting can arise quickly, so you might want to become aware now of the practical aspects of organization. Conventions and large-scale meetings require complex advance planning. But even the smallest sized meeting—two people—can be improved with some forethought. In your personal notebook, try briefly describing three or four topics that deeply interest you, along with a few questions or ideas you would like to explore. Then select one that could be a basis for a meeting. Try outlining a meeting plan using the following guidelines.

Purpose

Why should you hold the meeting? Think about the various things you wish to accomplish in the meeting. Is the purpose to discuss various points of view on a topic and then reach a decision? If the meeting is with one other person, is it to plan a collaboration? To share techniques or strategies? If it is with a large group, is one of the purposes to introduce new members of an organization to veteran members? Is it to hear a speaker or a special presentation? Is it to plan an event and list each member's responsibilities? Is it to evaluate and then plan to improve something? Are you trying to solve a problem?

To hold a purposeful meeting, you should first be able to describe how each person will benefit by being present. Some meetings begin with a statement of purpose to keep participants focused on the task at hand.

When possible, circulate announcements and any needed background material to participants before the meeting. This helps people to come better prepared and saves valuable meeting time.

The best meetings encourage people to interact, develop ideas, and plan activities based upon a clear theme or purpose. Meetings generally provide a forum to present ideas with opportunities for discussion or other ways for participants to respond.

Suppose the purpose of the meeting is to share ideas with the members of your photography club about entering a new photo contest. To prepare, you make a list of important items to list on the agenda. You will want to note the application, categories, entry fees, judging criteria, and deadlines. You will also want to share the contest rules and allow time for discussion. You may want to divide the group into smaller groups to discuss entry categories and the feasibility of some or all members entering. To close, you may want to get a commitment from those who plan to enter and agree on a process for submitting entries for approval from the club sponsor before mailing. Thinking ahead of time about what needs to be accomplished within the timeframe of the meeting will help you plan all aspects of the meeting.

If the purpose is simply to give announcements or routine dissemination of information, this is better done through a newsletter, mailbox flyer, or a phone message, rather than a meeting. People attending a strictly routine informational meeting may resent it, particularly if they feel they can use their time more profitably elsewhere.

Planning

You may benefit from the advice of someone who has had previous experience with the process of planning meetings. Pre-planning and thinking about the purpose will enhance the meeting results. Here are some additional planning questions to consider:

- How much notice must participants receive?

- What would be the best date? Will any holidays or other activities conflict with this date?

- Will facilities, needed materials, and speakers be available at this time?

- If a planning committee is needed, will the committee members have enough advance planning time?

- Is the meeting set up to allow reasonable amounts of time for each item on the agenda?

- Will someone be needed to take minutes of the meeting?

Participants

When planning a meeting, take a few minutes to consider who should attend. If the meeting is large, perhaps nametags would be beneficial. Also, if the meeting will be long, you may want to provide refreshments. A few more questions to think about include:

- Who should be there?
- How can they be notified?
- How can you find out who will attend, and later, who did attend?
- How will attendees benefit?

Publicity

Depending on the size of the meeting and the audience you want to attract, any of the following publicity approaches may be used: printed flyers, public address announcements, radio announcements, newspaper listings, printed or handmade posters, and/or press releases to news or print media. Consult someone with a background in journalism or marketing for the format to be used for press releases. You may be able to obtain sample press releases from other organizations.

Publicity should include the title of the event, date, time, place, cost, and sponsor, if applicable. Including a map or directions to help people locate the meeting place might be useful as well. If you are using posters or signs, check with officials to make sure that your approach is acceptable.

Agenda

An agenda should be prepared for every meeting. It could be just for your own use or passed out to all participants. In preparing the agenda, ask yourself what would make you want to attend the meeting.

If the printed agenda is something that all attendees of the meeting will see, make it interesting by experimenting with size, shape, color, format, and content. Encourage participants to refer to it during the meeting, especially if the agenda is complex. At the very least, it will afford people a place to jot notes and/or doodle.

Facilities

Where will you hold your meeting? Are you sure the meeting place will be available at the time you want your meeting to occur? Select a place that is large enough and easily accessible for the participants. Seek out free facilities by checking public and semi-public institutions. You may need the help of a committee and the advice of a mentor for large meetings. Publicize travel arrangements, such as car-pooling and parking facilities. Keep in mind any equipment or materials needed, such as a TV/VCR-DVD player or a flip chart.

Problems

Be aware, ahead of time, of health and safety needs. Pre-plan substitute activities. Key people may be late to the meeting. Speakers may fail to arrive. Some meetings—or items on the agenda—may suddenly become impossible because of unexpected events. Decide ahead of time about contingency plans.

Perfection is a rarity. When things go wrong, accept it as a challenge. Do the best that you can and remember to relax, smile, and enjoy your meeting.

Finale

The conclusion of every meeting should contain an opportunity to assess its value. Often this is done informally by briefly summarizing the meeting and asking for comments by the participants. Formal meetings featuring speakers frequently end with the distribution of evaluation sheets. If this is done, allow adequate time for their completion, collection, and review.

Write thank-you letters to guest speakers, sponsors, committee chairmen, and all who made contributions. If the news media were involved and were especially cooperative, make a special effort to express your thanks.

Arrange for a follow-up debriefing by a smaller group of participants. Ask the group members what actions should be the next steps after the meetings and how such meetings might be improved in the future.

Keep records of the meetings that you attend or arrange. What worked? What irritated? How could you improve upon the design?

What did you learn? How did you grow? What can you accomplish as a result of this meeting? When will you begin? Tomorrow?

Summary

- Meetings significantly affect human affairs.

- You can be an initiator of meetings.

- By following a guideline, the practical organization of meetings can be more effective and enjoyable.

Words of Wisdom

Management by objectives works if you first think through your objectives. Ninety percent of the time you haven't.
— Peter F. Drucker

A chairman of a meeting is like the minor official at a bull-fight whose main function is to open and close the gates to let the bull in and out.
— Dewey F. Barich

Few people know how to hold a meeting. Even fewer know how to let it go.
— Robert Fuoss

Having served on various committees, I have drawn up a list of rules: Never arrive on time; this stamps you as a beginner. Don't say anything until the meeting is half over; this stamps you as being wise. Be as vague as possible; this avoids irritating the others. When in doubt, suggest that a subcommittee be appointed. Be the first to move for adjournment; this will make you popular; it's what everyone is waiting for.
— Harry Chapman

The future is that time when you'll wish you'd done what you aren't doing now.
— Mary H. Waldrip

Use what talents you possess; the woods would be very silent if no birds sang there except those that sang best.
— Henry Van Dyke

To know oneself, one should assert oneself.
— Albert Camus

What we call results are beginnings.
– Ralph Waldo Emerson

When you go to meetings or auditions and you fail to pre-pare, prepare to fail. It is simple but true.
– Paula Abdul

If you had to identify, in one word, the reason why the human race has not achieved, and never will achieve, its full potential, that word would be "meetings."
– Dave Barry

People say, "So many meetings, no results," but no, that's not the point. Having so many meetings gives you comfort with each other and you are able to exchange views frankly, you are able to know each other better.
– Sellapan Ramanathan

To get something done a committee should consist of no more than three people, two of whom are absent.
– Robert Copeland

Chapter 14

Public Speaking: Doh! Do I Have To?

Fear of public speaking—whether it is in front of a class or at a meeting—is a source of anxiety for many people. Jerry Seinfeld once said that at a funeral, most people would rather be in the casket than to have to give the eulogy. But public speaking is an essential skill, even though it is not widely taught to students in schools.

The most famous of all Greek orators was Demosthenes 📖, a noted politician. He not only developed exceptional rhetorical skill, but he also became known for his use of simple and appealing language. Although he lived from 383 to 322 B.C., many of his speeches are still available today and have influenced modern orators.

Essence of Good Public Speaking

The essence of good public speaking is having something worth saying and saying it well and with great care. Proficiency in doing this develops with practice. Some families set aside one mealtime a week for speech practice. Each member, on a rotating basis, selects a topic, prepares a five-minute speech, delivers it, and then directs the subsequent dinner conversation. If possible, try this, or try it with a group of friends.

Imagine that you have been asked to speak to a class gathering or at some other meeting. Perhaps you have won an award and are to be honored, or perhaps you have been selected to speak at a school assembly. What an honor! What excitement! But how do you prepare? Enter the pertinent data—time, date, and place—into your personal calendar. Put reminder notes on the calendar at suitable intervals, such as two weeks before and one week before. Next, try to determine the needs and character of the audience. Why are you being asked to speak? If you are unclear, ask the person in charge. Discuss details carefully when the invitation is issued. How much time will you have to speak? Who will be in the audience? Is the purpose of the talk to inform, persuade, entertain, or a combination of these?

Once you have established the purpose, you should, of course, consider what exactly you plan to say. Try to anticipate what questions the listeners might have, and provide answers as you write your speech. Edit your material to fit the appropriate time. At a comfortable speaking rate, a six-minute speech would require about three double-spaced typewritten pages—or two minutes per page.

Check Your Content for Clarity

Remember, the audience probably knows less than you about this subject. There is a critical balance between saying too much and saying too little. Audience rapport tends to dwindle as a speech grows longer. It is better to leave your audience wanting more than wishing you had spoken less. In an informal speech, you can use audience reaction as a gauge of need for more or less detail.

A formal speech should be practiced for critique in front of people whose advice you value. If it is not feasible to practice your speech in front of a live audience, perhaps you can use a large mirror and a video camera or tape recorder set near you to record yourself. While being recorded, watch yourself in the mirror as you speak. How do you look? What kind of mannerisms do you have? After you finish, review the recording. How do you sound? Do you speak in a monotone, or do you vary your intonation? Are you animated? What detracts from your ideas? Do your gestures match the points your words are saying? What needs to be changed? Which of your comments seemed most useful?

Consider Your Style of Speaking

An interesting speech will alternate between generalities and specifics, between large views and detailed pictures. This pictorial analogy is appropriate because you will want to present your listeners with pictures through your words. Television and movies depend on "technical events" to retain audience interest. These include changes in camera range and perspective. In a speech, reasonable transitions from the overview to the details have a similar effect.

Build Suspense During Your Talk

For example, at some point ask a question that you do not immediately answer. Throughout your speech, provide additional insights until the answer becomes almost obvious. Then let the audience discover it. Or you can incrementally describe an unknown and then identify it as a climax. Or begin with impossibility and gradually turn it into a possibility. Work out other variations if this approach appeals to you.

Use Language Creatively

Alternate simple language with the richness of an anecdote or an allegory. Use the stimulating image found in a good metaphor. Develop clarity and impact with examples and analogies. You will be appealing to the creative thought processes of your listeners. View your speech as a gift package of your best ideas, wrapped in colorful language and presented with enthusiasm.

The bimonthly journal *Vital Speeches* is an excellent resource of recent speeches by people with established reputations in many fields, including politics, business, education, the arts, medicine, science, and law. These speeches can be examined for their technique, as well as for their contemporary thinking on a wide range of topics. You will probably find certain styles that are more impressive, and these are the ones you want to emulate.

After Your Speech Is Written

Once your speech is written, then what? If you will be speaking for a long time, you may want to use a triple-spaced, large-print copy completely edited with the exact wording that will be presented. You might underline or highlight key phrases or perhaps write reminders to yourself to pause, look at the audience, etc. If your speech is less formal or shorter, bringing a list of words or ideas, sequential file cards containing major points, or a partial copy of the text containing any unusual enrichments (examples, metaphors, etc.) may be sufficient.

If a speech must be presented verbatim, do not completely read it to your audience. Try to memorize substantial parts of it. Look up as often as possible to establish eye contact with your audience. Pause frequently at key points during your speech. Fluctuate the loudness and emphasis of your voice. A monotone sound will bore your audience.

Often the best speeches are extemporaneous, wherein the accidental interplay between audience and speaker creates a kind of magic. One idea leads to another so that even the speaker arrives at a mental destination previously unknown. Hopefully, this will happen to you at least once.

Whatever you can do to increase audience response and participation will be appreciated. Therefore, you may choose to build openings for audience participation into your speech. Ask the audience to do something at a subsequent point, perhaps to raise their hands or to speak a key word or phrase.

Will you be using an overhead projector or PowerPoint presentation to help illustrate your speech? If so, you will want to select the key points of your speech to be listed as bulleted points on the screen. You may also want to select images that will illustrate your points.

Using props or visual images during your speech will make people savor and remember what you have said. Creatively think how you might use ordinary objects to highlight or exemplify parts of your speech. For example, choose a speech topic and then see if you can figure out possible ways to use the following as props:

- A giant cardboard clock face with moveable hands.
- A mirror.
- A holder for large block letters plus extra letters.
- A balloon.
- Large sheets of drawing paper, an easel, and thick crayons.
- A wrapped package.
- Hats.
- A hammer, a nail, and a board.

After you are finished preparing your speech, you are still not done. Think about what you will wear on the big day. Choose comfortable clothes that are appropriate for the circumstances. Normally, avoid anything that looks bizarre or overly flashy or revealing. These kinds of fashions prevent the listeners from looking where they should be looking—at your face. Your clothes should permit simple, graceful movement. Tight or poorly fitted outfits create a poor image of you. And don't forget to wear comfortable shoes.

Speech Preflight Check

On the day of your speech, you have a few things to do before your big moment. Check all needed supplies and equipment before your departure. Leave enough time to arrive a bit early to double-check the arrangements. Make sure that you can use the microphone, if it is provided. Have someone listen to you from various spots in the room to ensure that you are neither too loud nor too soft. Quickly test all of your audio-visual materials.

If you are nervous before your speech, take a few deep breaths to calm down. When you are being introduced, remember that the audience will initially focus on your physical appearance. They will assess both your clothing and body language. Perhaps you will be tempted to bolt out of a chair, grab the lectern, and rush into a torrent of words. Or maybe you slump as you walk toward the center of the stage, clear your throat, gulp, and with head bowed, read rapidly from a sheaf of papers that audibly rustle. Resist these tendencies. Instead, hold your head high, briefly acknowledge the introduction, and smile. Eye-sweep the audience with a face retaining some vestige of that smile, and then proceed to speak.

If your movements are sharp and your papers shake, indicating your nervousness, don't worry too much; remember, audiences forgive and soon forget. Slumping, however, is a body language symbol for having no authority, and the audience will tune you out. A bowed head bounces sound into the podium, not out into the room. Stand tall with your head up!

Remember why you are speaking. Your ideas are being thoughtfully assessed by your audience. But if ideas alone were important, simply circulating a flyer would suffice. Speaking is a personal encounter. Therefore, you must, with all of your inner resources, project an image that demands attention and gains credence for your ideas. Partly, you do this with an animated face. Look at the people. With a large audience, use eye sweeps—scanning slowly front to back, side to side. Occasionally stop and appear to speak directly to one person.

Focal Points While You Speak

As you begin your speech, check that the most distant group of people can hear you by using someone as a spotter with prearranged signals. Be similarly sensitive to problems with ventilation, noise, heat, and light. Uncomfortable people cannot listen accurately.

Your voice is very important. Irritating voices—high-pitched, nasal, whiny, raspy, whispery—are tuned out by the audience. Imagine that you are speaking to a very dear friend, and let your voice develop appropriate warmth. Changing tone and pitch makes subsequent words more important (this wakes up the audience). Avoid singsong accenting of words because it irritates most people. A rise in pitch at the end of a sentence ("upspeak") makes you sound uncertain of what you are saying. Practice should permit you to attain reasonable pacing. Aim for a rate of about 150 words per minute.

If stage fright suddenly overwhelms you, pause and briefly contract your stomach muscles; keep them as tight as possible, then relax. Dr. Rozakis, in the *Complete Idiot's Guide to Public Speaking*, suggests: "Breathe from your diaphragm (your stomach) and through your nose. Don't breathe through your mouth." Look at one person in the audience, picking the friendliest possible face, and then keep going. The long-term best cure is practice. Eventually you will forget about yourself and become immersed in your speech. Stage fright disappears.

At the end of your speech, close with a summation. If audience response has been invited, prepare to think fast. Answer questions as you are able, but also admit ignorance when you must. Try to diplomatically handle anyone who heckles you or attempts to monopolize the floor. As you close your remarks, remember to thank the audience, your sponsors, and all of the on-stage personnel. Where appropriate, send a written thank-you note afterward to the person who invited you.

After Your Speech

A few days later, reflect on your speaking experience. How successful were you? How much did the audience respond? How could you improve? Maybe you will discover that you are a born speaker!

Try practicing these ideas by planning a speech on changes needed in your school or community. Summarize the results in your personal notebook.

Summary

- A good speech contains worthwhile ideas and is presented in a way that enhances the acceptance of those ideas.

- A good public speaker not only has a meaningful message, but also delivers it well.

- People can learn to be good public speakers, and public speaking improves with practice.

- A skillfully prepared content, a wisely projected personality, and a sensitive response to the audience will ensure success.

Words of Wisdom

There is nothing in the world like a persuasive speech to fuddle the mental apparatus.
– Mark Twain

The finest eloquence is that which gets things done.
– David Lloyd George

We live in an age of words, of talk, of constant oral expression. Language is getting progressively looser. Oral expression is sometimes graphic, but is often flabby. It is almost always repetitive. Nobody can speak quite as well as he can write, certainly as well as he ought to be able to write if he doesn't tie himself into knots of affectation.
– Erwin D. Canham

I have just got a new theory of eternity.
– Albert Einstein
(on listening to a long after-dinner speech)

Churchill wrote his own speeches. When a leader does that, he becomes emotionally invested with his utterances.... If Churchill had had a speech writer in 1940, Britain would be speaking German today.
– James C. Humes

Eloquence is logic on fire.
– Lyman Beecher

A speech is like an airplane engine. It may sound like hell, but you've got to go on.
– William Thomas Piper

There are three things to aim at in public speaking: first, to get into your subject, then to get your subject into yourself, and lastly, to get your subject into the heart of your audience.
— Alexander Gregg

According to most studies, people's number one fear is public speaking. Number two is death. Death is number two. Does that sound right? This means to the average person, if you go to a funeral, you're better off in the casket than doing the eulogy.
— Jerry Seinfeld

There are always three speeches, for every one you actually gave. The one you practiced, the one you gave, and the one you wish you gave.
— Dale Carnegie

A speech is poetry: cadence, rhythm, imagery, sweep! A speech reminds us that words, like children, have the power to make dance the dullest beanbag of a heart.
— Peggy Noonan

Political speeches are like steer horns. A point here, a point there, and a lot of bull in between.
— Alfred E. Neuman

Chapter 15

Determination and Persistence: Overcoming Obstacles and Difficulties

If the "how to" for achievement of goals could be summed up in three words, those words would be "perseverance," "determination," and "persistence." These are characteristics shared by all successful people throughout history. Of course, anyone can achieve easy goals with little effort or determination, but you want to set your goals higher than that. When you set your goals high, you are likely to encounter obstacles and difficulties, and that is where determination and persistence become important. How good will you be at holding firmly and steadfastly to your purpose, goal, or undertaking, despite obstacles, warnings, or setbacks? Will you have the mindset that will allow you to reach definite conclusions and be resolutely determined? Here are some ideas to help you.

Putting Ideas into Practice

Occasionally you may be so inundated with ideas that you can't find enough places to put them. Write them down so you can sift through this mental richness to find the good ideas—the ones that can be made to work. It is often said that ideas are cheap, but transferring ideas into practice is not, precisely because it requires effort, and all labor has a price.

If you *enjoy* thinking things up, you get an E for that kind of effort. When you can conceive of ways to implement ideas, you advance to a C grade. When you begin to convert ideas to action, you earn a B grade. When you actualize ideas, making them useful to others, you deserve an A grade. The latter requires persistence, and thus it is more highly valued. True persistence is uncommon; it has aspects of a devouring passion.

Just like the spider that must try many times to anchor a web, the inventor works long hours to succeed. Both have determination. You, too, have the ability to function productively, but how do you develop the required determination? By assuming that you will be successful. Visualize success! Whenever difficulties arise, return to this positive image. Then schedule work time, organize materials, and begin. Do not try to solve everything mentally apart from physical productivity. Commit your ideas to paper, canvas, or other reproducible entity. In writing, your ideas are sharpened; in painting, your visions materialize reshaped; in making something, your hidden problems and advantages modify original concepts. Even the tiniest success feeds determination. Problems that develop become your incentive to find solutions.

You may be working at the edge of technical possibility because you may need something that doesn't yet exist or exists unknown to you. Talk to people, research the literature, and send out letters of inquiry. This is no time to freeze; try to do something.

Work intently. A natural tendency is to wander off-target into distractions. Pencil tapping, a finger itch, thirst, or pleasant daydreaming interrupt constantly. Discipline yourself by practicing to minimize these distractions. Arrange the physical nature of your surroundings with this in mind. For example, some people like to have a window near their desk to look out of while thinking. Others may be distracted by what is outside and need to keep focused by putting their desk against a wall.

Finally, cultivate a stubborn streak. Refuse to quit. You may need to stop for a while, take a vacation, or pile up new resources. Start afresh, but don't give up!

Achieving Under Pressure

Sometimes things need to be done within a certain timeframe. Many practical strategies can help you achieve under pressure. Set up a schedule that permits certain checkpoints—what you expect to have completed at particular times. Make realistic estimates and then add, as a safety factor, a little extra time. Consider the following schedule selected by a writer:

The final draft must be ready by Tuesday, checked for grammar and sense by Wednesday, and a final copy must be produced by Thursday.

Problems with this schedule may occur. Perhaps some of the article ideas require considerable effort to develop, and the time that the writer allotted for writing becomes insufficient. Deadline pressures may result. Three solutions to this problem could be employed:

1. Delete nonessential activities to spend more time on the project.

2. Get a fresh start with a new idea to help the writing flow more easily.

3. Write an alternate article with an easier topic as a substitute.

If meeting a deadline is important to you, you might consider using one of these techniques—time shuffling, a fresh start, or substitution—since they are often applicable when troubles arise. Regardless of the option chosen, persistence toward the goal is key.

How you handle deadline pressure, or any other pressure, is vitally important. You can best do this if you have a strong belief in your ability to cope, can respond sensibly to reality, are able to manage no matter what, and can responsibly accept pressures as a fact of life rather than as a form of persecution. Instead of thinking, "Why does this always happen to me?" begin realizing that life would be less interesting without challenges. Anne Morrow Lindbergh describes a useful inner harmony in her book *Gift from the Sea*: "But I want first of all—in fact as an end to these other desires—to be at peace with myself. I want a singleness of eye, a purity of intention, a central core to my life that will enable me to carry out these obligations and activities as well as I can."

That last phrase—"as well as I can"—is important. It can prevent the "paralysis of perfection." When you fear being foolish or making a mistake, and therefore fail to act, you are making the most foolish mistake of all—namely, failing to accomplish what is possible. This does not mean that you should be satisfied with whatever you can produce minimally. But it does mean that *your best* is good enough.

When starting a project, you cannot know the final outcome. Snags may develop. For these occasions, use creative thinking processes. Sometimes a mini-vacation helps. Close your eyes and take a mental journey; fantasize. Listen to music. When you really feel grim, picture your past successes. Imagine future success. Get up and walk around. Look out the window. Sort through mentally stored images—perhaps randomly. Look at whatever objects lie before you. Then, since problems don't usually solve themselves, go back to work. You may find reading *Peace of Mind* by Joshua L. Liebman useful. Use your determination to succeed as a tool for getting the job done—and done well.

Meeting Deadlines

When your deadlines are set by other people, try to understand clearly what steps will be involved. Realize that written statements, clear descriptions, and contracts about deadlines are desirable, not only to have a record of the agreement, but also to clarify expectations from others who may not share your way of thinking. If their expectations differ from yours, try to think the problem through from their point of view, even though this may be difficult.

If you have accepted a deadline, try to meet it honorably. Do the best you can. Since it is true that work tends to fill the hours allocated, you may find that limits actually improve your output. However, if you find you cannot meet a deadline, address the problem *immediately*. Ask for a postponement; get help; do something! Failure to act responsibly is the only real mistake. Learn from the experience. Separate this particular failure from a self-failure label. *You* are not a failure; you simply failed at doing *this*. People who try can fail. People who fail have a chance to learn. People who learn from their mistakes succeed.

Be aware of procrastination. It is the opposite of persistence, and it affects many people. For example, you may have friends who are habitually late. They over-schedule themselves or become too involved in what they are doing or are simply delayed leaving on time. In response, you try to compensate for their tardiness by setting an earlier-than-necessary time for them to meet you, in the hope that they will actually arrive on time. Although friends may make allowances for tardy habits, other people may be less accommodating.

If you are frequently late or fail to meet deadlines appropriately, you may want to evaluate how you might modify these habits. They can affect your ability to achieve and to enjoy life. Consider why you are a procrastinator. Think about how you might change. On the next occasion that requires a timely response, make an all-out effort to meet this challenge. Don't abuse yourself if you fail. Just steadfastly persist. Several of these successes help you form a desirable habit.

Appreciate Patience

Patience is a virtue—and sometimes a pain in the neck. There is a human tendency to expect too much too soon because the mind leaps ahead. However, the spirit must endure all the barriers and indignities that occur along the way. You may be a naturally impatient person. If so, choose work that yields quick satisfaction, and do not embark on a 50-year breeding program for shade trees! If you are at the other extreme, capitalize on your patience. Recognize the fact that it is a valuable trait, and select work that requires it. However, beware of excesses. The overly patient person may not realize when something is useless or no longer valuable. Conversely, the impatient person may hot-headedly quit before reaching goals. Either extreme can limit you from reaching your potential.

What is the difference between persistence and patience? Persistence implies a more active pursuit and continuous effort. Patience allows for time lapses between effort and results or permits nearly repetitive trials to reach a particular result. Both are valuable in living a balanced life.

Summary

▣ Determination and persistence get the job done.

▣ Time pressures can be creatively managed.

▣ Habits of procrastination can be changed with effort.

▣ Patience and impatience affect your use of time.

Words of Wisdom

Knowing trees, I understand the meaning of patience. Knowing grass, I can appreciate persistence.
　　　　　　　　　　　　　　– Hal Borland

When I keep putting something off, it may not be procrastination, but a decision I've already made and not yet admitted to myself.
　　　　　　　　　　　　　　– Judith M. Knowlton

Procrastination is like a credit card: it's a lot of fun until you get the bill.
　　　　　　　　　　　　　　– Christopher Parker

In my youth, I stressed freedom, and in my old age, I stress order. I have made the great discovery that liberty is a product of order.
　　　　　　　　　　　　　　– Will Durant

There is a time to let things happen and a time to make things happen.
　　　　　　　　　　　　　　– Hugh Prather

Studies indicate that the one quality all successful people have is persistence. They're willing to spend more time accomplishing a task and to persevere in the face of many difficult odds. There's a very positive relationship between people's ability to accomplish any task and the time they're willing to spend on it.
　　　　　　　　　　　　　　– Dr. Joyce Brothers

I am personally convinced that one person can be a change catalyst, a "transformer" in any situation, any organization. Such an individual is yeast that can leaven an entire loaf. It requires vision, initiative, patience, respect, persistence, courage, and faith to be a transforming leader.
　　　　　　　　　　　　　　　– Stephen R. Covey

Never let your persistence and passion turn into stubbornness and ignorance.
　　　　　　　　　　　　　　　– Anthony J. D'Angelo

The difference between the impossible and the possible lies in determination.
　　　　　　　　　　　　　　　– Tommy Lasorda

The reasonable man adapts himself to the world; the unreasonable one persists in trying to adapt the world to himself. Therefore all progress depends on the unreasonable man.
　　　　　　　　　　　　　　　– Georg Bernard Shaw

I love deadlines. I like the whooshing sound they make as they fly by.
　　　　　　　　　　　　　　　– Douglas Adams

Tomorrow is the only day in the year that appeals to a lazy man.
　　　　　　　　　　　　　　　– Jimmy Lyons

Chapter 16

Health: Physical, Behavioral, and Mental

There is one absolute requirement for functioning as a human being—stay alive. A corollary concept is that your best functioning will probably occur if you can stay comfortably alive. But this can sometimes be a challenge.

You are a biological system made up of certain genetic codes and characteristics, some of which will probably remain unknown to you throughout your life. Some of these unknowns might be important hidden factors such as genetic defects or inherited tendencies for certain diseases. Another unrecognized influence could be the impact of the physical environment on your health—the possible long-term influence of even minimally contaminated necessities such as air, water, and food, as well as of the possibility of a sudden accident. A third factor is more directly controllable—namely your mental outlook, your attitudes, and your personality as they affect your lifestyle and ultimately your health. All of these factors—genetic inheritance, environment, attitudes, and behavior—must be managed to yield better health. But they can also be mismanaged.

Today, almost 60% of premature deaths are associated with behaviors or conditions that began or occurred during adolescence—for example, tobacco and alcohol use, poor eating habits, insufficient physical exercise, sexual abuse, and risky sexual behavior. Clearly, all of these can be managed, yet many people treat their personal health in a cavalier manner until threatened by some crisis. Often, they direct more effort toward maintenance of a car, or even a tennis racket, than toward self-preservation. On the other hand, too much concern with health, as exemplified by the activities of hypochondriacs, can also be counterproductive.

Consider the person who polishes a car daily, vigorously shining it. A shiny car is nice, but too much care can rub the paint away in what must certainly be an unintended result. Finding the right balance between carelessness and excess zeal is largely a matter of thoughtful experience. There are no simple guidelines to follow.

Self-Analysis

Knowing yourself will provide the best baseline for healthcare. Unfortunately, you were not born with a service manual, and therefore, you will have to "discover" yourself. You are unique, but you also have commonalties with your peers. By observing the experiences of others, you can develop useful insights for improving your chances of living a long and healthy life. As a suggestion, find time to be quietly alone occasionally, and use this time for self-analysis. What are you doing that is sensible? What can you change? Here are some questions to ask yourself:

- Do you eat breakfast every day?
- Do you eat at reasonable times during the day and consume reasonable portions?
- Do you maintain desirable body weight?
- Are you getting regular exercise?
- Are you sleeping seven to eight hours each night?
- Are you avoiding using tobacco, alcohol, and drugs?
- Do you abstain from or practice safe sex?
- Are you taking care of yourself emotionally?

Following these rules can not only dramatically increase your life span, but also makes the quality of your life more enjoyable. Statistics strongly support the value of these sensible and simple rules. Many physicians and psychologists now note that behavioral factors such as these are the most important health factors facing people today and are ones that people can control themselves.

Physical Health Problems

Although health issues are far more extensive than this book can cover, there are some problems that are particularly common for adolescents. For example, many people suffer from headaches. Certain headaches can be very serious and require immediate medical attention, such as headaches increasing in intensity over a period of hours or days, headaches followed by a fever having no discernable cause, headaches accompanied by mental confusion, or headaches following any blow to the head. One excellent source of information on headaches is the book *Heal Your Headache* by Dr. David Buchholz.

Many headaches, annoying but not as threatening as those mentioned above, are physical responses to stress or emotional problems. These include migraines, tension headaches, sinus headaches, and depression headaches. Dr. Buchholz describes people likely to have migraine headaches and gives concrete suggestions. Headaches can be debilitating—they prevent full functioning. If they are an affliction, you need to learn techniques to manage or heal them.

Another frequent health problem for adolescents is stomachaches, many of which also stem from stress. The concept of stress management has wider application than that of controlling headaches or stomachaches. Many years ago, a French psychotherapist, Emile Coue (1857-1926) 📖, advocated healing by optimistic autosuggestion. A typical self-affirming statement of this approach was, "I am getting better and better every day in every way." The mind and body are very much interrelated, and psychologists and psychiatrists sometimes treat a physical disease by using mental suggestion.

Eating disorders, including anorexia and bulimia, can be very serious and are often found in persons who are sensitive, perfectionistic, rigid, and have great pride in their accomplishments, but yet have feelings of anger or resentment. Sometimes behaviors such as eating disorders, headaches, or stomachaches arise because a person is trying to suppress hurt feelings, perhaps because of physical or sexual abuse that he or she has experienced or witnessed. It this is your situation, it would be wise to talk to a professional, or at least a trusted adult.

Perhaps the most widespread physical health problems for adolescents come from behaviors such as smoking, drinking, drug use, risky sexual behavior, and reckless or angry outbursts. Homicide, suicide, and auto accidents are the three leading causes of death among adolescents and young adults. Our sexualized society, combined with peer pressure, can make it tempting to engage in risky behaviors of drinking, drug use, and sex. However, these can have long term, and even fatal, consequences.

Illnesses can be physical manifestations of emotional problems, stress, and nervousness. Attempting to cure or ameliorate physical symptoms without addressing their cause seldom produces lasting results. Therefore, learning how to manage your emotional state is at least as essential to your continued health as finding a good doctor.

Behavioral and Mental Health Problems

Some behavioral and mental health problems may be even more important for you to consider because of your capabilities. For example, you may feel that there are not enough hours in the day for you; you simply cannot fit everything in to the time you have available. It is exciting and wonderful to be able to do so many activities and to be so intensely involved. However, when people are preoccupied with many pressing tasks, they may be accident-prone because of their preoccupation, because they are doing things too quickly, or because they are tired from so much effort and perhaps too little sleep. The resulting accidents may lead to injuries. Thus, under time-stress conditions, you may need to be particularly alert to managing potential behavioral health issues.

You probably have a love of exploration and may enjoy being the first to try, to do, to see. You may even like to live "on the edge." There is a strong likelihood that you are often successful in these ventures and greatly enjoy them. Initially, you may be blessed with beginner's luck, or you may triumph as a result of cautious planning and intelligent effort. The health-operative word here is "cautious." Exploration can be very hazardous. People who function at the edge of the unknown must be nimble of foot and wit to survive. Some do not survive. The lucky ones try again.

Multiple successes can lead to a kind of fatigue carelessness. Precautions take effort, and eventually making the effort seems to be unessential when nothing bad happens. The chemist fails to use a safety shield for the hundredth time because nothing happened during the proceeding 99 times. The explorer seeking new plant material in the Amazon jungle fails to check the snake bite supplies on his hundredth expedition. Guess what happens. Success can also lead to thinking that you are invincible. You think that you can instantly solve any problem because you know that you can solve many challenges easily. Caution does not imply that you need to retreat from the joys of exploration, only that you need to set out carefully *every time.*

Pay attention to clusters of accidents, such as breaking or losing things, falling, or bumping into things. These may be signals of unresolved stress. Some introspection may be helpful if this is the case. Identifying stressors and then eliminating them from your life will not only make you happier, it will actually increase the amount of time you have for doing the things that excite you, as opposed to searching for lost car keys or nursing bruised shins.

Other behavioral or mental health problems arise from intense and often disturbing feelings. Particularly common are feelings of depression and loneliness or of not being understood. Everyone occasionally feels angry, frustrated, sad, depressed, worried, lonely, or uncertain. However, when these feelings persist and impair your normal functioning, you may need to see your doctor. Symptoms that may indicate the need for professional help include persistent moodiness, irritability, changes in appetite, sleeplessness, preoccupation with high-risk activities, intense concerns about physical appearance, or withdrawal from friends and family. Talk to a relative, teacher, counselor, or family doctor. The essential beginning to getting better is the willingness to admit to having a problem, then being determined to overcome it with help.

Many behavioral and mental health problems are common, well understood, and treatable. Your family doctor may be able to refer you to a local counselor or therapist. There are many kinds of psychological therapies, such as psychoanalytic, behavior, cognitive, person-centered, group, and counseling. Choosing suitable help takes knowledgeable effort. An excellent library reference source is *The American College of Physicians Complete Home Medical Guide.* This book has many informative sections on physical and mental illnesses. It also includes extensive online sites for many health agencies in the United States, such the American Psychological Association, at www.apa.org, and the National Mental Health Association, at www.nmha.org/index.cfm.

Even quite serious mental illnesses can be treated very successfully when properly recognized. One, for example, is manic-depression, also called bipolar disorder. Among the famous people who likely had this disease are George Fredrick Handel 📖, Antonio Rossini 📖, Robert Schuman 📖, Honore de Balzac 📖, Vincent van Gogh 📖, Ernest Hemingway 📖, Theodore Roosevelt 📖, Winston Churchill 📖, Joshua Logan 📖, and Patty Duke 📖. Symptoms of this affliction commonly begin in the late teens to early twenties. Diagnosis often is based on recording alternating extremes of moods and behavior that go from very high and elated to very low and depressed over a long period of time. This appears to be an inherited disorder, not controllable without medical help. An excellent book on the subject is *A Brilliant Madness: Living with Manic-Depression Illness* by Patty Duke and Gloria Hochman. Ms. Duke relates her personal experiences with great courage and honesty.

Change What You Can

You cannot change everything about you that you may want to change. The eminent psychologist Martin Seligman, Ph.D., examined the research and wrote a book titled *What You Can Change—And What You Can't: The Complete Guide to Successful Self-Improvement: Learning to Accept Who You Are.* Things that can be altered are patterns of thinking and acting, particularly thinking that leads to anger, depression, phobias, and anxiety. Traits more resistant to change—some may even be unchangeable—are sexual identity, post-traumatic stress reactions, and the tendency to be overweight.

The most advocated methods to prevent illness are dietary precautions, exercise, and elimination of the smoking habit. Obesity, which has become a national health problem, is related to lack of exercise. Our modern conveniences entice us to be passively entertained. It can be easy to sit in front of the TV or computer for long periods of time, but try to take activity breaks such as walking the dog or running around the block. It is important to eat thoughtfully rather than by habit or simple convenience. Balanced diets that are low in saturated fats and cholesterol are recommended.

Self-Improvement Suggestions

Because the mind and body interact, a healthy mind is directly related to a healthy body. Even though you may not see yourself as being flawed, you are likely to see potential benefit in some suggestions for self-improvement. These suggestions are not complicated. If fact, they are disarmingly simple.

- Smile.
- Make a conscious effort to really enjoy something each day.
- Slow down.
- Recognize that hostilities are a corrosive agent.
- Maintain interests in a wide variety of cultural activities.
- Actively seek to be with people.
- Listen.
- Avoid interrupting.
- Turn your attention to worthwhile tasks.

Your body has a tremendous range of physical, chemical, and physiological structures. And like other living organisms, change in these structures is part of being alive. As you mature, major changes take place. Some of these changes are obvious and external; others are subtle and internal. The world around you likewise is continually changing. Your mental and emotional responses to changes influence your activities and total being for the rest of your life.

Be kind to yourself when calamity strikes or when any major change affects your life. Death, illness, job loss or change, moving, loss of a friend, unusual success—all of these can be stressful events. You should have strong feelings and be capable of expressing them, accepting the help of friends whenever possible. Consider the probable psychosomatic origin of any sudden health problems that develop during times of change and stress, and share your suspicions with your doctor.

Value life and take care of yourself. Care about others, for that is one root source of a stable psyche. Refuse to yield to social pressures that can endanger you—no matter how persuasively expressed. This is particularly important because of the social use of drugs. Drugs (including alcohol) can be very risky and are directly and indirectly capable of causing irreversible damage to you, physically and mentally. Drugs are not necessary for expanding your mind. Any mind-altering should be accomplished by your conscious effort—not chemically induced. Recognize that health is related to the *quality* of your life—joyous, creative, and socially responsible.

Sexual experimentation can be extremely risky and have life-long health effects. Fortunately, you have the ability to choose how you want to behave. Of course, sexuality is important to life, but it is not the totality of your being, nor that of anyone else. Any problems or questions concerning sex should be discussed with responsible family members, a physician, or similarly trustworthy people.

Many sexual variations exist, just as humanity has variability in hair color, height, and facial features. Labels such as heterosexual, homosexual, and bisexual do not describe anyone completely and should not be a source of discrimination.

Your birthright includes your right to control your health so that you can live more joyously. Whatever may be your life span, your biological inheritance, or your daily circumstances, if you value *being*, you will be comfortably alive.

Describe your health—mental and physical—in your personal notebook. Repeat this process at regular intervals, perhaps annually, and think about any changes.

Summary

- ▣ You can manage inheritance, environment, and behavior to obtain better health.

- ▣ Awareness of your self is essential to any realistic health program.

- ▣ Adhere to a few common sense health rules to achieve longevity.

- ▣ Carelessness and overconfidence can lead to accidents.

- ▣ Psychological wholesomeness may be your most important resource in achieving good health.

- ▣ Whatever may be your particular circumstances of well-being, enjoy each day as it exists.

Words of Wisdom

The more serious the illness, the more important it is for you to fight back, mobilizing all your resources—spiritual, emotional, intellectual, physical.
– Norman Cousins

(Today's students) can put dope in their veins or hope in their brains. If they can conceive it and believe it, they can achieve it. They must know it is not their aptitude but their attitude that will determine their altitude.
– Rev. Jesse Jackson

Two out of every three deaths are premature; they are related to loafer's heart, smoker's lung and drinker's liver.
– Dr. Thomas J. Bassler

Brush them and floss them and take them to the dentist, and they will stay with you. Ignore them and they'll go away.
– American Dental Association

Coroners (they always have the final word) know why cocaine's nickname is killer.
– Dr. Joseph Pursch

There are no such things as incurables; there are only things for which man has not found a cure.
– Bernard M. Baruch

For me, the creative process, first of all, requires a good nine hours of sleep at night....
– William N. Lipscomb, Jr.

It is health that is real wealth and not pieces of gold and silver.
– Mahatma Ghandi

The health of the people is really the foundation upon which all their happiness and all their powers as a state depend.
> – Benjamin Disraeli

So many people spend their health gaining wealth, and then have to spend their wealth to regain their health.
> – A. J. Reb Materi

Health is a state of complete physical, mental and social well-being, and not merely the absence of disease or infirmity.
> – World Health Organization

When it comes to eating right and exercising, there is no "I'll start tomorrow." Tomorrow is disease.
> – V. L. Allineare

Red meat is not bad for you. Now blue-green meat, that's bad for you!
> – Tommy Smothers

Chapter 17

Mentors: Sources of Wisdom, Advice, and Experience

"It isn't what you know, it's who you know." This bit of folk wisdom is often true. If you collect contacts—people who can be helpful to you under special circumstances—the way other people collect knowledge of celebrities, you are being wise. A modern term for this process is *networking*.

One special relationship you should seek to establish is with a mentor. The word "mentor" originates from Greek mythology. Mentor was the friend of Odysseus 📖 who entrusted him with the education of his son Telemachus 📖. In modern parlance, a mentor is someone who is a trusted counselor, guide, tutor, or coach; a more experienced mentor helps a less experienced mentoree.

Many mentor relationships develop naturally. Our earliest mentors are typically admired family members who provide acceptable guidance while we are growing up. Other mentors may be teachers, family friends, neighbors, and employers. These relationships, even if they are short-lived, are often very influential. However, the most valuable mentorships usually develop as a result of careful thought and search. Think about what you wish to do. Think about your special interests. Who is likely to be knowledgeable in these areas and willing to share their expertise with you?

Locating a Mentor

Locating a suitable mentor will be a challenge, but there are some useful techniques that can help you. Once you have selected a general area in which you want to learn more, ask your parents or a friend of the family who they might be able to introduce you to. Most adults have established a network of connections and can help you make contacts. Though this may seem improbable to you, remember the "six degrees of separation" concept 📖—that is, no person on earth is more than six contacts away from any other person.

Perhaps you can locate someone with established professional status through descriptions of their activities in newspapers. Sometimes you can even obtain contact information for that person from the newspaper or the Internet. Often such people win awards, organize conferences, become officers in organizations, publish, exhibit, and generally obtain public recognition for their achievements. It may be possible for you to attend public events where they are present. Arrange to meet them, and try to make that meeting memorable. Write a follow-up letter expressing your interest in their work or ideas. Write a letter of congratulations for honors received, and include a brief account of your own aspirations. Ask for advice, and tell them you are looking for a mentor. You may be surprised to learn how accessible some such people are and how willing they are to become mentors.

Another source for locating a mentor is the Internet. National organizations such as Mentor (www.mentoring.org) and Icouldbe.org (www.icouldbe.org/standard/schools/schools_about_us.asp) match mentors with students. Their e-newsletters contain much useful information, and e-mentors represent hundreds of career paths.

Whether you find a mentor in your community or via the Internet, most people will be flattered by your request to have them as a mentor and may wish to help you. Of course, some of them will be reluctant to accept the responsibility and time commitment that goes along with being a mentor. Do not apply pressure. You are seeking wise counsel and asking that it be freely given to you. Be realistic in your demands. As an unknown—the apprentice, the person at the bottom—you cannot expect people who are very busy to expend much time on your behalf. Make your questions brief, be observant, and make your interest and appreciation apparent. Nourish any developing relationship by being thoughtful.

You may also find mentors through organizations that relate to your career interests and by becoming an active member. Accept committee work. Volunteer for tasks that will be shared with more experienced members. Do you admire someone? Ask them for counsel on appropriate occasions. When you find their counsel useful, tell them and thank them. When that experienced person voluntarily contacts you to give you suggestions, you will have found a mentor.

To maintain this relationship, you will need social skill. You should also think of what you could offer in exchange for the expertise shared and the connections supplied. Perhaps you could help your mentor with routine work, such as mailings. Perhaps you could offer to do some Internet searches. Your enthusiasm generally will make up for your lack of expertise.

A mentor can locate unusual sources of information, provide guidance in technique, introduce you to other helpful people, and smooth the way for you to accomplish more with less effort. To achieve a good mentor relationship, you need to be willing to reveal both your desires and your abilities. Even in a good working association, you may occasionally need to tactfully reject advice. After all, you must make your own decisions; your mentor cannot live your life for you. If you find yourself frequently rejecting advice, you need to carefully evaluate the relationship.

Mentors Can Help in Your Career Path

Being mentored may also help you in your career path. Suppose you have made a career choice but have no real idea of what that kind of work entails. Try to obtain employment in this area. It might just be a part-time job or an unpaid internship. Almost all professional fields are associated with supportive service jobs. Find one of these, and you can observe the professional work at closer range. These experiences provide you with a good chance to evaluate a potential career and possibly to find a mentor.

College students, including those high school students who take an occasional college course, have exceptionally good opportunities to locate a mentor. Professors usually are at the leading edge of knowledge within their field, enjoy sharing their knowledge, and are influential. Any extra time spent in their company provides you a chance to learn and observe. Some students offer their assistance, paid or unpaid, in research endeavors just to obtain mentor benefits. Some of these relationships result in life-long personal and professional relationships.

When you ultimately become employed, you may need to know that many companies expect their professional personnel to make use of mentors. You may be assigned to someone who becomes your guide and guardian. If you can choose your mentor, do so with a long view toward advancement. By alignment with someone "on the way up," you can achieve a coattail effect and rise too.

Friends as Mentors

Mentoring can arise casually from friends sharing experiences. One friend is an experienced traveler and helps you plan vacations to exciting places. Another friend shares her expertise on theatrical events. Someone else becomes a guide on personal fitness. But you may at some point feel the need for new horizons to explore—a change in the focus of your leisure life.

You may want to develop a planned approach to expanding the range of people who can influence your life using some of the same techniques suggested for obtaining career mentors. Seek people who seem to have a special "joie de vivre," or joy of life. You may be able to establish an assembly of people from many backgrounds—including art, politics, science, young and old, rich and poor, like-minded and contentious—all able to socialize well. Such a group might meet infrequently, with its structure and existence mutually established.

A classic example of this is Contesse Marie Jeanne DuBarry (1743-1793) 📖, who established a famous court circle, or *salon*, of artists and literary people. Similarly, Alexander Woollcott (1897-1943) 📖 was the leading member of the Algonquin Round Table, which met in the 1930s in the Algonquin Hotel in New York City. Members of his group included Harpo Marx (comic/actor) 📖, Robert Benchley (actor, drama critic, and writer) 📖, Dorothy Parker (writer) 📖, George S. Kaufman (playwright) 📖, and others.

Undoubtedly, many groups of a similar nature exist today. Perhaps the pleasant exchange about human experiences (informal mentoring) is a concept that you could explore. Certainly, there have been many famous people who benefited from being mentored. For example, in the entertainment field, Gwyneth Paltrow 📖 was mentored by Madonna 📖, and Johnny Carson 📖 mentored Jay Leno 📖. In sports, Patrick Ewing 📖 mentored Alonzo Mourning 📖, and Phil Jackson 📖 mentored Michael Jordan 📖. In music, Isaac Stern 📖

mentored Itzak Perlman 📖, and dance star Martha Graham 📖 mentored Agnes de Mille 📖.

Finally, whenever you can, become a mentor yourself. In the simplest sense, share what you know as freely as possible.

Summary

▣ Mentors can help you accomplish more with less effort.

▣ There are opportunities throughout life for the development of mentor relationships.

▣ Selecting mentors requires creative effort and social skill.

▣ Being a mentor is a worthwhile experience.

Words of Wisdom

A good teacher has been defined as one who makes himself progressively unnecessary.
— Thomas J. Carruthers

No matter what accomplishments you achieve, somebody helps you.
— Althea Gibson

If you would thoroughly know anything, teach it to others.
— Tryon Edwards

If you have knowledge, let others light their candles at it.
— Margaret Fuller

To teach is to learn twice.
— Joseph Joubert

A great teacher never strives to explain his vision—he simply invites you to stand beside him and see for yourself.
— Rev. R. Inman

Only a life lived for others is a life worth while.
— Albert Einstein

He that won't be counseled can't be helped.
— Benjamin Franklin

Mentor: someone whose hindsight can become your foresight.
— Anonymous

Successful people turn everyone who can help them into sometime mentors!
— John Crosby

My values and beliefs were imparted to me by loving parents, committed teachers, demanding mentors and wise elders.

– Jesse Helms

I was lucky that I met the right mentors and teachers at the right moment.

– James Levine

You know, at various times in my career, I've been fortunate enough to have hooked up with some fantastic mentors.

– Rob Lowe

The biggest difference is in the leadership. It was better for us. We had more coaches and mentors to help us. A lot of the younger players today suffer from a lack of direction.

– Isiah Thomas

Chapter 18

Success: What Is It, Really?

The limousine stalled just before the lift bridge. As the chauffeur endeavored to find the trouble, the grey-haired passenger emerged and strolled toward the little shack of the bridge-tender.

"What a surprise! What are you doing here?" he asked.

The man in the shack looked up from his book and slowly replied, "Reading." His tiny wooden table was cluttered with books, scraps of paper, and the remains of a paper bag lunch.

The visitor, looking closely at the bridge-tender, asked, "Do you remember me? Weren't we classmates at Yale?"

The bridge-tender nodded in agreement.

"Then why are you here?"

"It gives me the time to do what I enjoy most of all—read." With this reply, he went back to reading his book—oblivious to the shock on the face of this visitor.

Who do you think made better use of his education or his life? Who is more successful? Why? Can you really tell from such a simple account? Does it matter?

Success is one of the magic words of modern society. There are commonly accepted standards of success, but there is also an aura of private meaning. It is this personal meaning that tends to become our lifetime guide. You will need to set your own goals if you want to have a focus. As the saying goes, "You have to name it to claim it." This is the first stage toward achieving success.

Take time to reflect on what success means to you. You might do so by completing each of the following statements, either below or in your personal notebook.

1. Among my immediate acquaintances, _____ is most successful because _____
   _____.

2. Among the famous contemporaries known to me, _____ is most successful because _____
   _____.

3. Among all historically famous people known to me, _____ was the most successful because _____
   _____.

4. I'll feel successful today if _____
   _____.

5. I'll feel successful this week if _____
   _____.

6. I'll feel successful this year if _____
   _____.

7. At the end of my life, I'll feel successful if _____
   _____.

8. To be successful, I need to _____
   _____.

Did you find answering the questions challenging? Was it difficult to select successful people? How did you react to thinking about your own success? What were your feelings as you read the vignette at the beginning of the chapter?

The nature of success can be ambiguous. Think of the bridge-tender and the man in the limousine. One person's success is another person's failure. You can develop your own concept of success—what it is, what it is worth, and how to achieve it. You can't examine success quite as easily as you can study a leaf or a stone, but you can apply some of the same principles of scholarship. In fact, if you answered the questionnaire, you have begun the process.

The second phase of studying success could reasonably involve surveying the literature.

The following descriptions of some "success" books may be useful for you. You will find them to be interesting reading.

1. *Skills for Success: A Guide to the Top for Men and Women*, Adele M. Scheele, Ph.D. (1996). Dr. Scheele's book is inspirational; it describes career competencies that would be useful in many areas, and it makes success an ethical imperative. In-depth interviews with Ely Calloway 📖, Dom DeLuise 📖, John Brooks Fuqua 📖, and Shirley Hufstedler 📖 provide illustrations of Dr. Scheele's premises.

2. *Ambition: The Secret Passion*, Joseph Epstein (1989). Mr. Epstein provides an intellectual voyage through America's history, highlighting it with short biographies of illustrious Americans. The epilogue is especially interesting.

3. *The Arc of Ambition: Defining the Leadership Journey*, James Champy and Nitin Nohria (2001). These authors describe the styles and contributions of three kinds of leaders: creative visionaries, capitalizers, and consolidators.

4. *Molloy's Live for Success*, John T. Molloy (1984). The author offers practical advice on his specialty—appearance—as well as on functioning at job interviews, public meetings, and in various office situations.

5. *The Power of Intention*, Dr. Wayne Dyer (2005). The author explores the psychological basis for success in great detail. Many of Dr. Dyer's ideas mesh with those in Dr. Scheele's book, even though the perspective is different, and success in a traditional sense is not the main topic.

6. *What's Holding You Back?: 8 Critical Choices for Women's Success*, Linda Austin, M.D. (2001). Dr. Austin provides professionally derived insights into the achievement process for women. Although this practical information is especially useful for women, it is also valuable for men who share the working world.

7. *Success is a Choice: Ten Steps to Overachieving in Business and Life*, Rick Pitino with Bill Reynolds (1998). Using many examples from his experience as a basketball coach, Mr. Pitino develops 10 specific techniques for achieving success. This motivational approach is easy to read.

8. *The Seven Habits of Highly Effective People*, Stephen R. Covey (2004). This work, a probable classic in the literature of success, contains elegant assessments of a principle-based approach to achievement. A must-read book.

9. *The 7 Habits of Highly Effective Teens*, Sean Covey (2003). Sean Covey writes from the point of view of a teenager, and this book has practical advice on improving one's self-image, building friendships, resisting peer pressure, achieving goals, and getting along with parents while searching for success.

10. *The 7 Habits of Highly Effective Teens Personal Workbook*, Sean Covey (2003). A thought-provoking workbook with interesting exercises to help teens make better decisions and practice habits that will make them more effective in achieving their goals.

11. *Life Strategies: Doing What Works, Doing What Matters*, Dr. Phil McGraw (2006). This is an intensely personal examination of how people can view and assess themselves, others, and life in order to achieve goals, happiness, and success. This realistic study of 10 significant common characteristics of people is accompanied by interesting examples of behavior.

The third phase in your scholarly study of success is to actively pursue a course of action. You can't just talk the talk; you have to walk the walk. Why not try it? Write a book, a paper, or a poem. Paint a picture. Write a sonata. It might not be perfect product, but if you finished it, then you have succeeded! List some successful people you would like to know more about in your personal notebook. Follow up with information you discover concerning one of your choices.

Here are some helpful tips toward finding success:

■ Start where you are, look around at what you have and what you can use, and launch a dream. No place is too small to begin.

- Consider the probable requirements for the type of success you desire. Can you realistically meet them?

- Work hard, not in isolation, but in the context of a richly varied and sometimes supportive human community.

- Take calculated risks. If failure occurs, learn from it and proceed.

- Develop patience with uncertainty, imperfection, and ambiguity?

- Consciously, and sometimes subconsciously, use your knowledge and experiences to cultivate yourself. Learn and grow.

- Be responsible and concerned for others.

- In the long run, honesty always pays.

- Plan ahead. For example, don't rush from one traffic signal to the next. Use timing and alternative routes.

- The classic advice "Find a need and fill it" usually works.

Summary

- Success can mean different things to different people.

- You need to develop your own definition of success and then pursue it earnestly.

- There are many good books available that offer advice on how to find your own personal success.

- You can't succeed if you don't try.

- Be eager to accomplish, rather than to simply garner awards or rewards.

Words of Wisdom

My mother drew a distinction between achievement and success. She said that achievement is the knowledge that you have studied and worked hard and done the best that is in you. Success is being praised by others, and that's nice, too, but not as important or satisfying. Always aim for achievement and forget about success.
— Helen Hayes

Success is that old ABC—ability, breaks, and courage.
— Charles Luckman

No one can possibly achieve any real and lasting success or "get rich" in business by being a conformist.
— J. Paul Getty

Pick battles big enough to matter, small enough to win.
— Jonathan Kozol

The tragedy of life doesn't lie in not reaching your goal; the tragedy lies in having no goal to reach.
— Benjamin E. Mays

If I have been of service, if I have glimpsed more of the nature and essence of ultimate good, if I am inspired to reach wider horizons of thought and action, if I am at peace with myself, it has been a successful day.
— Alex Noble

Strive not to be a success, but rather to be of value.
— Albert Einstein

I haven't failed. I have successfully discovered 12,000 ideas that don't work.
— Thomas Edison

Success means having the courage, the determination, and the will to become the person you believe you were meant to be.
> – George Sheehan

Don't wait until everything is just right. It will never be perfect. There will always be challenges, obstacles and less than perfect conditions. So what. Get started now. With each step you take, you will grow stronger and stronger, more and more skilled, more and more self-confident and more and more successful.
> – Victor Mark Hansen

To laugh often and much; to win the respect of intelligent people and the affection of children...to leave the world a better place...to know even one life has breathed easier because you have lived. This is to have succeeded.
> – Ralph Waldo Emerson

Success means doing the best we can with what we have. Success is the doing, not the getting; in the trying, not the triumph. Success is a personal standard, reaching for the highest that is in us, becoming all that we can be.
> – Zig Ziglar

The road to success is always under construction.
> – Lily Tomlin

Real success is finding your lifework in the work that you love.
> – David McCullough

Chapter 19

The Landscape of Courage: Resilience over Rocky Terrain

The landscape of courage is uneven. Life inevitably will contain moments of fear, but your quick strokes of strength can help you meet these challenges with competence.

It is the management of everyday life that nourishes the roots of courage. Getting up, getting going, and getting to use—not abuse—each day takes courage. It takes inner strength to push outward, be with people, pursue tasks, make decisions, live with the results of those decisions, loosen ideas into the public domain, have those ideas judged, learn to perform, and be tested. It is easier sometimes to stand still, be a child, be cared for, withdraw, and do the minimum. It is truly awful to watch the parade pass by from a hole in the ground—to so limit extension and involvement that the viewing-eye level is on the pavement.

There is a "blood, thunder, and glory" version of courage. Its usual source is fear—physical or social—so intense that adrenaline flows and action is possible. Revolutionaries, battle participants on war maneuvers, racecar drivers, and contestants of all kinds have a need for courage. This kind of valor can light up the sky with its intensity briefly, like firecrackers.

But courage is not limited to occasional feats of dramatic public risks such as saving someone's life. Actions under the white, hot glare of instantaneous need, such as pushing a child away from an oncoming car, are important fodder for newspaper headlines precisely because of their rarity. Though some rescue actions may be deliberately courageous, like those of firefighters, for instance, others may be almost reflexive, like the man who instinctively dives into icy water to save a girl from a submerged car without considering that he might be placing his own life in jeopardy. Some rescue responses may actually be acts of cowardice.

Instead, courage can be simpler and quieter, perhaps internal in nature. It takes courage to stand up for what you believe in if it goes against the grain of public opinion. It is courageous to admit mistakes and forge ahead to try again. Learning something new after having been comfortable with an old way of doing things takes courage. In all of these examples, courage is exhibited because someone stepped out into the unknown, oftentimes alone, and believed in the power of the self to weather the consequences.

There are no training institutes for courage, although one could argue that both the armed forces and sales training schools build toward it. There are no technical manuals that explicitly prepare you to be courageous. However, there are many inspirational books that treat courage as an important human trait. One example is *Find Your Courage!: Unleash Your Potential and Live the Life You Really Want* by Margie Warrell. This book describes practical ways in which you can become more courageous in your everyday life and how you can embrace the challenge of reaching for your potential.

But knowing what courage is does not automatically make one courageous, just as reading about chocolate is not the same thing as tasting it. Is there any day when courage is not needed? Is today your day to taste courage? Will you meet the challenge?

> What is your attitude toward your own courage?
> You may be saying: "When the time comes, I'll be ready."
> You may be saying: "How will I know what to do?"
> You may be saying: "I'll never know until something happens."
> You may be saying: "Just try me."

Thomas Carlyle 📖 said, "Depend upon it, the brave man has somehow or other to give his life away." At face value, this implies that bravery is associated with risking death. But from another viewpoint, Carlyle could be suggesting that bravery is living so as to give away something of value to others, by creating, by accomplishing. By living to this extent, you give your life away—to a cause, to an art, to a person. Such living has a purpose that exceeds self-maintenance. It is valorous.

Every part of daily existence has some opportunity to be brave, take chances, and extend yourself. If you want to launch a courageous life, look within yourself and examine your personal beliefs; then act in accordance. President John F. Kennedy's *Profiles in Courage* describes instances of political courage. The last few paragraphs of the *Young Reader's Memorial Edition* of this book are worth remembering:

> *For, in a democracy, every citizen, regardless of interest in politics, "holds office"; every one of us is in a position of responsibility; and, in the final analysis, the kind of government we get depends upon how we will fulfill those responsibilities. We, the people, are the boss, and we will get the kind of political leadership, be it good or bad, that we demand and deserve.*
>
> *These problems do not even concern politics alone—for the same basic choice of courage or compliance continually faces us all, whether we fear the anger of constituents, friends, board of directors or our union, whenever we stand against the flow of opinion on strongly contested issues.... The courage of life is often a less dramatic spectacle than the courage of a final moment; but it is no less a magnificent mixture of triumph and tragedy. A man does what he must—in spite of personal consequences, in spite of obstacles and dangers and pressures—and that is the basis of all human morality.*
>
> *To be courageous...requires no exceptional qualifications, no magic formula, no special combination of time, place and circumstances.... In whatever arena of life one may meet the challenge of courage, whatever may be the sacrifices he faces if he follows his conscience—the loss of his friends, his fortune, his contentment, even the esteem of his fellow men—each man must decide for himself the course he will follow. The stories of past courage can define that ingredient—they can teach, they can offer hope, and they can provide inspiration. But they cannot supply courage itself. For this, each man must look into his own soul.*

There are probably some things that you are sensibly and rightly afraid of, and other things that you are foolishly and unreasonably afraid of. There are life-preserving fears, such as fire, falling, or drowning. There may also be inhibiting fears, such as meeting people, taking tests, or public speaking. Regardless, knowing how to handle your fears is useful. Is there a method or strategy that works?

You have to push open your own door to find the landscape. The latchkey may be hard to find, and the opening may be small. But once you step away, you won't want to stop. And almost nothing will stop you.

Write a brief account of the most courageous act that you have ever witnessed in your personal notebook. Add other occasions as you discover them, and review them periodically.

Summary

- ▣ Courage is essential to thoughtful daily living.

- ▣ Collective acts of courage have made civilization possible—even for the cowardly.

- ▣ The habit of courage can be internally programmed.

Words of Wisdom

All serious daring starts from within.
– Eudora Welty

The time when you need to do something is when no one else is willing to do it, when people are saying it can't be done.
– Mary Frances Berry

Everyone has talent. What is rare is the courage to follow the talent to the dark place where it leads.
– Erica Jong

Courage is very important. Like a muscle, it is strengthened by use.
– Ruth Gordon

Courage is doing what you're afraid to do. There can be no courage unless you're scared.
– Edward V. Rickenbacker

Give me the serenity to accept what cannot be changed. Give me the courage to change what can be changed. And the wisdom to know one from the other.
– Reinhold Neibuhr

I have had dreams, and I have had nightmares. I overcame the nightmares because of my dreams.
– Jonas Salk, M.D.

The courage to imagine the otherwise is our greatest resource, adding color and suspense to all our life.
– Daniel J. Boorstin

Why not go out on a limb? Isn't that where the fruit is?
– Frank Sailly

It takes a lot of courage to release the familiar and seemingly secure, to embrace the new. But there is no real security in what is no longer meaningful. There is more security in the adventurous and exciting, for in movement there is life, and in change there is power.
— Alan Cohen

Moral cowardice that keeps us from speaking our minds is as dangerous to this country as irresponsible talk. The right way is not always the popular and easy way. Standing for right when it is unpopular is a true test of moral character.
— Margaret Chase Smith

If you lose hope, somehow you lose the vitality that keeps life moving, you lose that courage to be, that quality that helps you go on in spite of it all. And so today I still have a dream.
— Martin Luther King, Jr.

Courage without conscience is a wild beast.
— Robert G. Ingersoll

If my mind can conceive it, and my heart can believe it, I know I can achieve it.
— Jesse Jackson

A ship is safe in harbor, but that's not what ships are for.
— William Shedd

It is curious—curious that physical courage should be so common in the world, and moral courage so rare.
— Mark Twain

Chapter 20

Social Etiquette: Traditions, Customs, and Rituals

The incredible richness of brain functioning in humans supports an equally rich and complex structure of behaviors and interactions with others. Every society establishes its culture through various traditions and rules about how people speak, act, and even think. These customs—which don't always seem to make sense—are the glue that holds groups, society, and even our families together. It is important to understand human behavior so that you can be more comfortable in complex social interactions, feel at ease socially, and help others feel the same way. Probably the best way to achieve this degree of behavioral comprehension is to develop your ability to think consistently of the needs and desires of others.

Your ability to sense the thoughts, attitudes, or feelings of another person is called empathy; it is the human trait most responsible for soothing the stresses of human interaction. Reading body language, assessing a tone of voice, and noting mannerisms helps everyone respond with better awareness to other people and allows our interactions to flow smoothly. All of this is a part of what has been called emotional intelligence 📖.

Good Manners

Successful diplomats and politicians usually have extraordinary empathetic skills. The words polite and politician share common Greek and Latin word origins. Richard Gephardt's book, *An Even Better Place: America in the 21st Century*, presents cogent arguments concerning how to make political structures more effective. He states: "Thus, mutual respect and civility among members of Congress aren't merely desirable; they are the only practical basis upon which our government can be run."

Unfortunately, just wanting to do the right thing and really caring about others may not be enough. Often we must know the elaborate rules for various social occasions that exist within our society. Although most rules of social etiquette reflect common sense attitudes about the best ways for people to interact, some rules may appear to be ridiculous or irritating. Some of the silly ones are remnants of behaviors needed in the past. Many of the present male-female rules, such as pulling out a woman's chair for her, are of this type. Other customs, such as focusing on how a person speaks and the grammar used, are maintained to identify class members—upper, middle, and lower. Communities and groups also tend to develop certain customs that are useful in identifying "belongers." For example, people at social gatherings observe—often unconsciously—the actions of people whom they have not met; their observations will determine whether they decide to be friends or whether they will let certain individuals remain strangers.

On occasion, you may break the social rules, whether knowingly, carelessly, or possibly as a result of ignorance. When you do, others around you usually will have negative reactions. You have suddenly become unpredictable and have challenged the status quo. As a penalty, they may subsequently exclude, avoid, or try to limit you. At first glance, social rules may seem stifling. Surprisingly, though, living by the rules generally tends to permit more personal freedom than would occur by ignoring rules.

On the other hand, sometimes social customs need to be challenged. Remember, for example, the longstanding traditions in the Deep South concerning segregation, or the custom of denying women the right to vote or hold political office. Even now, discrimination exists in ways that are unfair, yet are customary. You may decide to confront and defy such customs, but know that there will always be a price to pay, because these types of actions will make other people uncomfortable and possibly even angry.

In many social situations, you will need to learn to do a cost-to-benefit analysis. That is, you'll need to determine whether it is too expensive or ineffective to challenge outdated traditions, and then weigh what the benefits might be of not challenging. In other words, pick your battles. Is this really a dispute that would be worth it? Is there a less confrontive way of achieving your goal?

Become an Observer

How do you learn social rules? Become an observer. Emulate people who have good social grace; analyze successful and unsuccessful situations, and use your insights to develop sensible and sensitive behavior. Good manners can defuse tense situations. Also, concern for another person's point of view tends to produce a reciprocal effect. A smile, a handshake, and pleasantries about family or circumstances can make any social event better for both you and others.

The Written Word

In an age of easy verbal communication, the promptly written thank-you note has a special cachet. Assemble a stationery folder and fill it with an assortment of notepaper, cards, and stamps. Correlate the quality of your stationery with the circumstances of its use. Then write as often as possible—to express gratitude, congratulations, acceptance, a point of view, etc. Skill develops with practice. There are entire books on how to write letters for most occasions. The important thing to remember is that letter writing is not only a valuable art, it is a necessary adjunct to desirable social behavior. Appropriate social behavior is important to the work culture of many organizations.

With today's electronic methods for communicating, however, many people may be tempted to correspond exclusively by means of e-mail, instant messaging, and text messages. While this may be acceptable for normal day-to-day interactions, it is still preferable to send written letters or notes as a way of expressing thanks, sympathy, and more. In fact, your willingness to take the time to handwrite a note will make you stand out above the crowd in our increasingly technological—and therefore impersonal—society.

Be Willing to Abide by Etiquette

You may be judged critically at some important point in your life on what may appear to be a nonsensical set of rules—namely, table manners. Consider what is meant by being *willing* to abide by etiquette. For example, there is no absolute functional necessity for placing forks tine-side-down on your plate when you have completed a course. It does, however, provide a silent signal to the waiter. It marks you as being a knowledgeable person and a conformist in an area where conformity has little or no philosophical overtones, but rather has a practical communication value. Thus, observance of table manners and other rules of etiquette provide a clue to character and intelligence and can also make events more positive than they otherwise might be.

A bit of "when in Rome, do as the Romans do" often applies to the social scene—there must be a reasonable matching of behavior to the circumstances. Otherwise, you may unintentionally be offensive.

Rudeness

If good manners are the balm and lotion of human society, then rudeness is the sandpaper. Not that rudeness is without value. There may be occasions when deliberate rudeness is useful—but such occasions are very, very rare. For example, Anne's friend Tara constantly interrupted her, even when others were present. Anne would begin, "Next Thursday, I think we should..." and Tara would interrupt, "Why next Thursday?" Initially, Anne tried humor, as well as both gentle and firm direct requests to Tara to stop her irritating habit—all ineffective. Finally, Anne succeeded, though it required a firmness that was somewhat rude. At a small committee meeting, Anne's words were cut off as usual. Then Anne spoke loudly and with slow emphasis, "Since Tara knows what I am going to say before I do, I think that she is capable of doing my work before I do. Therefore, I vote that Tara be assigned to both write the notices and make all of the telephone calls. All agreed? Good. Motion carried." Tara for once was speechless.

You do not, however, want to be rude unintentionally. Is there a possibility that you sometimes are unwittingly offensive to others? Even your best friend may be unwilling to tell you that you have unpleasant mannerisms. Interrupting a speaker, being inattentive, not returning letters or phone calls, toying with table implements, rocking on dining chairs, putting feet on furniture, snapping gum (or chewing it publicly), monopolizing conversations, not returning greetings, forgetting to say thank you, not meeting obligations, and failing to treat *each* person as you would wish to be treated—all of these habits are abrasive and deleterious to your social success.

Attend to the Little Things

Attend to the little things, for it is often the small behaviors that describe and give color and flavor to human nature. Thomas Jefferson 📖, in designing Monticello 📖, made the staircases very narrow—too narrow to permit comfortable passage for any woman in the wide skirts of that time. The implication is that he did not act considerately with respect to the needs of the women in his household. In many other instances, especially when entertaining guests, he was a thoughtful person. Flaws are a part of human nature. You should try to eliminate your own flaws as they become obvious, but do not expect perfection. Thomas Jefferson was an exceptional statesman, a creative architect, and a much-admired host, but he was not perfect.

Sometimes friction arises because you expect others to act in a certain way, but they may have different ideas. It is likely that a simple communication problem exists, but other explanations are possible as well. Your expectations may be unrealistic; they may, in fact, be impositions. For example, you may expect Jarell, because he is your best friend, to take care of your dog while you are on vacation. You explain how to feed and exercise the dog and when you will be back. When you return, you find a jubilant pet but a resentful friend who cancelled other opportunities because of his duty to your dog. From this point onward, your friendship deteriorates. Why? Jarell was very busy and didn't have the time to take care of your dog, but he hadn't been candid enough to say no because he was trying to be a good friend. For someone else who had more free time, your expectation would have been reasonable. You need the sensitivity to discern the difference or to ask in such a way that your friend could say yes or no comfortably.

Gratitude

With practice, you will have fewer occasions of interpersonal friction and more pleasant relationships where good manners are present. Often, such smooth interactions will result in gratitude. However, two ideas concerning gratitude are particularly valuable. One, do not expect gratitude—*ever*—or you may find yourself feeling like a beggar who is rattling a tin cup in vain. Instead, do things simply because they are good and need to be done, not because you expect a reward. Two, express your gratitude to others whenever possible. It is amazing how few people remember to convey appreciation, even though a simple "thank you" is very powerful.

To put these ideas in perspective, consider your own experience. Have you thanked everyone who made a special effort on your behalf? If not, why not? Did you secretly carry your feeling of gratitude? That is very normal. Now think about occasions when you helped others but did not receive any recognition for your efforts. That, too, is very normal. But how did you feel? Did you feel encouraged to continue and to do more, or were you discouraged?

A straightforward verbal thank you such as, "I appreciate the time you gave me," a note of appreciation, or a spontaneous return of a favor are welcome responses to favors received. Let your sensitivity extend to everyone who affects your life—not just those who are powerful or important or who might give you special treatment. Imagine that you are the other person, and respond accordingly. Put yourself in the other person's shoes.

Begin today if this is not already your method of interaction with others. People will be delightfully surprised, and your own life will be richer. Finally, one additional valuable aspect of gratitude is its ability to nourish excellence of behavior. By telling someone that you appreciate what is being done, you provide encouragement for them to continue that behavior.

Of all the multitude of possible behaviors, how often have you selected behaviors that were good etiquette? What about your future choices? Record your thoughts on your social behaviors in your notebook.

Summary

- ▣ Learn and use the rules of etiquette.

- ▣ Manners are the foundation of social interaction.

- ▣ Careful observation of people can lead to improved social skills.

- ▣ Deliberate rudeness can be desirable on occasion.

- ▣ Confer gratitude frequently, but expect it rarely, if at all.

Words of Wisdom

Do good to thy friend to keep him, to thy enemy to gain him.
— Benjamin Franklin

Rudeness is the weak man's imitation of strength.
— Eric Hoffer

Civility costs nothing and buys everything.
— Lady Mary Wortley Montagu

Life is short, but there is always time for courtesy.
— Ralph Waldo Emerson

And so, my fellow Americans: Ask not what your country can do for you—ask what you can do for your country.
— John F. Kennedy

Behold, I do not give lectures or a little charity—when I give, I give myself.
— Walt Whitman

Love your enemies, for they tell you your faults.
— Benjamin Franklin

Each day comes bearing its gift; untie the ribbons.
— Anne Ruth Schabacker

Good manners will open doors that the best education cannot.
— Clarence Thomas

One of the greatest victories you can gain over someone is to beat him at politeness.
— Josh Billings

Don't reserve your best behavior for special occasions. You can't have two sets of manners, two social codes—one for those you admire and want to impress, another for those whom you consider unimportant. You must be the same to all people.
— Lillian Eichler Watson

Nothing is less important than which fork you use. Etiquette is the science of living. It embraces everything. It is ethics. It is honor.
— Emily Post

Tradition is a guide and not a jailer.
— William Somerset Maughan

Chapter 21

Ambition's Gamble: Finding a Rewarding Career

Finding a rewarding career is a worthy ambition. Careers are not the same thing as jobs, though jobs are a component of careers. A career is a lifelong pursuit, one that hopefully you will enjoy and can feel passionate about.

Employment can supply the necessities of life, some luxuries, a source of self-esteem, and an opportunity for creative expression. The parameters of each of these possible outcomes derive, in part, from your ambitions. At various times in your life, you may seek work just to earn money, with little regard for the learning that can take place or the satisfaction value of a good job. Summer jobs and part-time work are often examples of this kind of employment. But a career search usually is undertaken with greater care because you are attempting to satisfy a larger range of needs. You have to understand yourself and your ambitions to make career choices. What do you know about seeking employment? How do you intend to satisfy your ambitions?

Seeking Employment

Getting a job can be like assembling a complicated object with the aid of an enclosed diagram. The diagram looks simple, the parts are simple, but at first, they just don't go together. Eventually, though, persistence pays off and the assembly occurs. The same thing can happen in seeking and keeping employment.

In the job market, your personality may influence the way you go about searching for a job. If you are shy and introverted, you might decide to simply send your resume to companies or to use the services of an employment agency. If you are social, good at sharing, and someone who enjoys personal involvement, you might decide to phone companies for more information or seek out people who work there. If you are extroverted and assertive, you might decide to call the company and directly request an appointment to discuss job opportunities.

The following accounts briefly detail the work experiences of six very talented, but very different, young people. As you read them, think about your own circumstances.

Fred found a summer job working as a gardener's assistant. He showed up for work on the first day with a radio and hung it on a nearby tree. It blasted out rock music, startled birds, and ruined neighborhood tranquility. Fortunately, he was perceptive enough to leave it home the next day—or he would have lost a job which he came to enjoy deeply.

Rafael couldn't get any summer work locally but obtained a job as a waiter in a distant summer resort. His neat and clean appearance, willingness to work hard, and good humor impressed several influential guests. He not only accumulated enough money through tips for his first college semester, but he also made personal contacts useful for future employment.

Upon graduation from high school, Tamika found a job as a receptionist/typist in a small office near her home. She felt trapped and bored within two months.

After carefully surveying his aptitudes and desires and obtaining appropriate college training, Roy went into the computer repair business for himself. He is now president of a company at the leading edge of a growing industry.

Almost through high school and uncertain of career direction, Amelia feels a bit frightened. Part-time work in her chosen field of cosmetology has been unsatisfactory.

Making use of talents in several areas, Christine has become an author and has achieved a high-ranking job in the banking industry.

For your first job, people older than you are likely to do the hiring; therefore, sensitivity considering their attitudes and values probably will be essential to becoming employed. Fred's use of the radio, while acceptable and sensible from his point of view, was offensive and unreasonable to his employer. Even a good worker, if irritating, will eventually be fired. Appearance, mannerisms, and speech habits can affect employment. Employers judge employees both by outward appearance and by what they can accomplish.

Both Fred and Rafael made good use of their summer earnings. In each case, they obtained college degrees. They did something else, too—they did some learning on the job. They learned how to work, even if it was hot, tiresome, or downright unpleasant. Fred developed an avocational interest in nature when he decided that birdsong was worth listening to and floral patterns were incredibly varied. Perhaps these patterns will one day subconsciously affect his work as an architect. Rafael learned how to listen to people, to please them, and to make them notice him. He developed talents that would later help him become a widely respected lawyer. Every job has potential for self-education. To gain the most from a job, act in such a way that your education and your employer's needs are not in conflict.

Compared to Fred and Rafael, Tamika carefully planned and prepared for her first job. She felt confident that just being employed and receiving a paycheck would be a great experience. She would finally be able to buy her clothes without parental approval. Throughout high school, she resisted many suggestions from her teachers that she take college entrance courses. She was very intelligent, but the problem was that her family would not support her going to college. Neither of her parents had gone, and they had each obtained jobs out of high school which they worked at for many years, both earning a decent income. Therefore, they felt that Tamika would be wasting money on an education when she could be making money instead.

Tamika lacked enough self-esteem and determination to seek work commensurate with her abilities. When her employer, who recognized her potential and was sympathetic to her situation, finally insisted that she go back to school on a part-time basis, she obtained her undergraduate college degree in five years. As a young researcher, she has already published a number of outstanding papers. The lesson here is that you could be stymied more by self-concepts than by realities. The best career preparation should be realistic in terms of your abilities, not your self-doubts.

Of these six people, Roy may seem to be the luckiest. He is his own boss. However, for most of the past 10 years, Roy's working days have been 12 to 15 hours long, and he has often worked seven days straight. Uncertainty and poor living conditions could have swamped his success, except that he believed in himself and really enjoyed what he was doing. His wife is a partner and professionally competent. By providing employment and services to many others, their efforts have greatly enriched their community. Presently, they can afford to take occasional vacations, and they maintain a luxurious home. But they paid their dues in terms of delayed pleasures. If you see yourself in the future as being self-employed, take note that it takes initiative, effort, and courage, but the rewards can be generous.

Amelia chose work that she found to be physically demanding, though mentally boring. Since almost any occupation can be turned into a creative outlet if you can see the possibilities, why does Amelia feel stifled? Her choice, cosmetology, could lead to product development, marketing, consulting, and writing; it need not be limited to beauty shop work.

Trial experiences like Amelia's may be unrewarding, but she can look for guidance from several sources—the Internet and the library. Some of the best books are very inexpensive; their purchase could be an excellent investment since you will likely refer to them frequently. The following books are especially helpful:

- *What Color Is Your Parachute? 2007*, Richard Nelson Bolles (2006). This is a highly acclaimed bestseller. The author is the director of the National Career Development Project. Before you commit yourself to any career direction or contemplate getting or changing any job, read this book. It clearly describes all of the practical details of obtaining a job—from interviews to resumes, from handling rejection to locating resources. Richard Bolles also publishes a bimonthly *Newsletter about Life/Work Planning*. Information about this is included in the book.

- *Occupational Outlook Handbook*, available from the Superintendent of Documents, Government Printing Office, Washington, DC 20402. Current price and availability should be checked. Most large libraries have a copy. This annual publication describes 300 occupational clusters with jobs in each cluster, including duties, requisite training and qualifications, potential earnings, and the prognosis for future employment.

- *Encyclopedia of Career and Vocational Guidance* (2007). This multi-volume resource provides information useful in identifying your abilities and talents. Again, it is likely to be found in large libraries.

Finally, consider Christine's multiple accomplishments. They are the output of an assured, highly intelligent person. Her experiences suggest that when one occupation fails to answer one's needs, it should be augmented with another outlet—a secondary activity. No one occupation carries the guarantee of being fully satisfying. In examining career choices, think of clusters of related activities that you might enjoy pursuing as a hobby. Also, think of combining interests when choosing a career. For example, interests in business, art, mathematics, and engineering could lead to selecting architecture as a career.

Whatever direction you choose, be a self-starter. Pick up your own two feet and point them somewhere. Do not depend on someone else to decide for you or to tell you what to do. Ask advice. Seek information. But make up your own mind. Everything that you do involves risk. If you do the selecting, you can best accept the results.

James A. Breaugh reported some pertinent findings in the *Academy of Management Journal.* He discovered that people who worked hard at uncovering job openings by using their own initiative were happier and performed better than those people who answered want ads or used various employment services. Why? Probably because their efforts gave them more accurate information about available jobs and thus made them less likely to take unsuitable work.

What do employers want? According to career consultants Randall and Katharine Hansen, the top 10 skills sought are:

1. Communication skills—the ability to listen, speak, and write effectively

2. Analytical/research skills—the ability to analyze a situation, gather key information, and identify issues

3. Technical/computer literacy—almost all jobs now require some basic understanding of computer hardware and software

4. Flexibility/adaptability—the ability to manage multiple tasks simultaneously, set priorities, and adapt to changing situations

5. Interpersonal abilities—the ability to relate to coworkers of various backgrounds

6. Leadership/management skills—the ability to create a productive climate that inspires coworkers

7. Multicultural sensitivity/awareness—an ability to develop and maintain rapport with persons of diverse cultural and ethnic backgrounds

8. Planning/organizing—the ability to set goals, identify details needed, and implement action

9. Problem solving/reasoning/creativity—the ability to creatively generate workable solutions to problems

10. Teamwork—the ability to build trusting and productive relationships with coworkers

In addition to skills, however, employers look for personal values in people who apply for employment. Here are the top 10, according to Hansen and Hansen.

1. Honesty/integrity/morality

2. Adaptability/flexibility

3. Dedication/high work ethic/tenacity

4. Dependability/reliability/responsibility

5. Loyalty

6. Positive attitude/motivation/energy/passion

7. Professionalism

8. Self-confidence

9. Self-motivation/ability to work with little supervision

10. Willingness to learn

CollegeGrad.com conducts surveys of leading employers, and in addition to the skills above, they note, "Passion about the opportunity is important to employers because it cannot be taught or faked. When employers recognize that a student's enthusiasm and excitement about the job is genuine, that student will most often get the job." Robert G. Traxel, author of *Manager's Guide to Successful Job Hunting,* long ago noted that what most employers "want—and hardly ever get—is a person with a gleam in the eye and a dream in the head." This has not changed. Can you measure up? To be ambitious is a gamble, but one where the potential profit is high.

Write a brief imaginary account of your ideal future employment in your personal notebook. How can you get there?

Summary

- Your interests and ambitions direct your occupational choices.

- Analyze your employment for learning opportunities.

- There are excellent resources available to use in career planning.

Words of Wisdom

Luck is a matter of preparation meeting opportunity.
  – Oprah Winfrey

No race can prosper 'till it learns that there is as much dignity in tilling a field as in writing a poem.
  – Booker T. Washington

The person who knows "how" will always have a job. The person who knows "why" will always be his boss.
  – Diane Ravitch

The two important things I did learn were that you are as powerful and strong as you allow yourself to be, and that the most difficult part of any endeavor is taking the first step, making the first decision.
  – Robyn Davidson

The secret of joy in work is contained in one word—excellence; to know how to do something well is to enjoy it.
  – Pearl S. Buck

One should labor so hard in youth that everything one does subsequently is easy by comparison.
  – Ashley Montagu

The work of the individual still remains the spark that moves mankind ahead even more than teamwork.
  – Igor Sikorsky

Make no little plans: they have no magic to stir men's blood.... Make big plans, aim high in hope and work.
  – Daniel H. Burnham

Life is to be lived. If you have to support yourself, you had bloody better find some way that is going to be interesting. And you don't do that by sitting around wondering about yourself.

– Katharine Hepburn

The difference between a job and a career is the difference between forty and sixty hours a week.

– Robert Frost

What is the recipe for successful achievement? To my mind there are just four essential ingredients: Choose a career you love, give it the best there is in you, seize your opportunities, and be a member of the team.

– Benjamin F. Fairless

I have frequently been questioned, especially by women, of how I could reconcile family life with a scientific career. Well, it has not been easy.

– Marie Curie

Don't ever let economics alone determine your career or how you spend the majority of your time.

– Denis Waitley

If the career you have chosen has some unexpected inconvenience, console yourself by reflecting that no career is without them.

– Jane Fonda

Chapter 22

Solitude: Alone or Lonely?

From the outside, solitude and loneliness may seem quite similar, but in fact, they are very different. Loneliness implies a negative feeling of being isolated; solitude is a state of being alone without feeling lonely. Solitude allows time for reflection, enjoyment, inner searching, and thinking.

Some of us feel compelled to be with others; we are afraid to be alone. Yet self-chosen solitude can be a delightful gift to yourself. You can let your mind wander into space, imagining, thinking, rehearsing activities, meditating, mentally concentrating upon a task intensely, or withdrawing into your inner being. No one speaks to you to interrupt your reverie. No one demands your attention.

Imagine that you are a potter, an artisan who works with clay to produce three-dimensional objects such as vases, bowls, and plates. Normally you share studio space with other artists, but on this particular day, you are alone. You pick up a chunk of wedged clay, enjoying the feel of its wet pressure and its smell, reminding you of garden soil after a rainfall. Then you remember a toy that you played with in your mother's garden. Your surroundings seemingly disappear as you concentrate on the potter's wheel before you. Your whole being centers on an idea that leads you to create an abstraction of that toy in clay.

When your friends see the final piece, they are surprised. You have "broken out of a mold," produced something that you had never before thought of—in a solitude intruded upon by physical sensations and memories. Did being alone enhance your creativity? Possibly, but even when no other person shared your space, you still had company—your human nature and its sociable extensions. Characteristically, people are sociable. In isolation, your thoughts over that prolonged period of time probably involved other people, other places, and other times. So you were never totally alone.

Finding Solitude

When you share living space with others, when you are almost constantly surrounded by people, the opportunities for solitude diminish. How do you find this "space?" By being inventive. Perhaps you can create opportunities by rearranging sleeping times. Turn a part of the night into day and vice versa. As a small child, you may have used bedsheets to create a cave for yourself under a table. Now you can seek privacy by taking a walk to some sheltered spot, finding a quiet corner in a library, or letting family know that your residence in a particular place means that you need to sometimes be alone.

Is your occasional desire to be alone selfish? In one way, yes, because it is a natural human quality to be concerned with who you are and who you want to be. In another way, no, because this quality time with yourself may help you become a better person, more sensitive to others, with a more fully developed conscious self.

As an exercise in self-development, try the following. In your first session, begin by doing as little as possible. Simply sit or lie down somewhere quietly for at least 10 to 15 minutes, though up to an hour is preferable. Close your eyes and, to the extent possible, "drown out" external sounds and sensory impressions. You may set an alarm clock to end the session if you must have definite closure. If possible, use a low volume music alarm to create a soft ending. Otherwise, let your inner spirit drift until you feel a need to stop. Then, after stopping, immediately record your "quiet voyage," using whatever means you prefer. Do this for succeeding voyages with the intent of discovering the merits of this process. This is a practice with an ancient lineage—a process of meditation.

Sometimes, in the magic moments of awakening from sleep, you may sense a fullness of being. Gradually, your conscious mind perks up, intrudes, and ideas start tumbling in rapid succession. These brief moments of solitude can yield exceptional and inventive answers to problems that have been a concern to you. You may wish to keep pen and paper or a recording device by your bedside to preserve these ideas while they are clear to you.

When Solitude Is Not of Your Choosing

There is another kind of solitude—a solitude that is not of your own choosing. You may occasionally feel isolated and alone because no one understands or accepts you. Perhaps you are not popular, or perhaps you are rejected even by people close to you, such as your friends or family. You reasonably resent this kind of solitude. It may be of brief duration, or it may become a long-term problem. What happens as a result of this solitude will depend upon your determination to achieve your dreams, your aspirations, and your acceptance of yourself (quite correctly) as a very special person.

How to Deal with Rejection

What should you do when you feel this kind of loneliness because of rejection? Although analyzing reasons for the problem may be helpful, such attempts may be governed more by feelings than by logic. Under stress, your insight into the actions of others may be flawed. Since you do not really know another person's reasons for rejecting you, you must guess. You may be incorrect, and even if you are correct, what then?

If you desire to change your circumstances, you must react. Getting angry is the least desirable reaction, because anger tends to beget anger. It is likely that you will only worsen the situation.

In contrast to the heat of anger, an icy cold withdrawal into yourself may occur. You may retreat, isolating yourself from almost all human interaction. This is also a mistake, even a tragedy, because everyone belongs somewhere within the vast panoply of humanity. All of your special qualities and talents will remain hidden and unshared if you withdraw. Here are some suggestions to help you deal with feelings of isolation:

- Realize that this is a common experience. Dr. Goleman states in his book, *Emotional Intelligence*, "the feeling of being rejected and friendless is one most everyone goes through at some point in childhood or adolescence."

- Try to develop a larger perspective and an optimistic attitude. The actions of a few do not represent all of humanity; you can turn your attention elsewhere to find acceptance.

- ◙ Actively seek the perspective of at least one sympathetic person (family member, teacher, doctor) whose opinions and judgment you value. Evaluate their advice carefully.

- ◙ Develop the ability to respond positively to others; take their occasional arrows and blunt them. Knowledge of human nature, known as psychology, is useful. The Internet is filled with information on psychology, and libraries and bookstores have numerous books on it.

- ◙ Make use of the calming effect of being outdoors. Go for a walk. Visit a park or a garden. This may be a source of inner peace and an antidote to interpersonal problems.

- ◙ Consider that perhaps the problem is not you and not others. Instead, examine whether it occurs because you are in the wrong place at the wrong time. If so, eventual changes will likely solve the problem.

- ◙ Develop proficiency in an activity that you enjoy and that is widely admired. You will probably meet people with similar interests who could become your companions and friends. As your proficiency develops, you will find that you win friends and that your feelings of aloneness will diminish.

One of the most inspiring humans who suffered incredible childhood isolation became a famous writer and counselor for the American Foundation for the Blind—Helen Keller 📖. Her disability of being blind and deaf as a result of a disease she suffered from when she was only 19 months old deprived her of all normal human communication until a teacher and friend, Anne Sullivan Macy 📖, was able to breach that terrifying silence. Eventually, Helen Keller learned to speak. She graduated from Radcliffe College cum laude in 1904 and subsequently received honorary degrees from universities all over the world. Many of her books tell of her early isolation and later triumphs. You may realize from this brief description of her achievements that her disabilities and involuntary isolation had positive results both for Ms. Keller and the larger world.

An extraordinary book by Prudence Kohl, *Hole in the Garden Wall*, with exquisite photographs, intensely personal essays, and poetry, contains a quote that is relevant here:

> *To be alone is a matter of choice;*
> *To be lonely is a matter of circumstance.*
> *One is a conscious decision;*
> *The other, a cry for help.*

Involuntary isolation can enhance the creative efforts of those determined to meet its challenge, even in this least joyous type of solitude. The cry for help is answered by one's own problem solving in many instances. For example, efforts by prisoners in isolation have included mentally improving a skill, such as playing golf or the piano, by imagining its performance over and over again. Even with no paper or laptop computer available, books have been written, mathematical systems invented, poetry created, and letters to loved ones constructed—all in the mind of the person. These coping mechanisms made the prisoners' confinement more bearable and less destructive to their humanity.

How can you use this information? Hopefully, you will never experience the solitude of imprisonment, abandonment, isolating illness, or physical disabilities. However, if any of these should occur to you, know that you not only can survive, but actually can creatively turn a limitation into an opportunity. You would have illustrious predecessors: Sir Thomas More 📖, Sir Walter Raleigh 📖, John Bunyan 📖, Fyodor Dostoevsky 📖, Ludwig van Beethoven 📖, Francisco Goya y Lucientes 📖, Henri Matisse 📖, Vincent Van Gogh 📖, Nelson Mandela 📖, and Stephen Hawkins 📖, among others.

During World War II, Dr. Victor Frankl was a prisoner in a Nazi concentration camp for years, during which he analyzed why some prisoners were able to survive, whereas others perished. After the war, he wrote his powerful book *Man's Search for Meaning In the 1980s*, journalist and political hostage Terry Anderson 📖 was able to survive incredibly harsh circumstances of isolation by using various mental means such as designing crossword puzzles, writing poetry, and mentally revisiting previous events. He describes his imprisonment experiences in the book *Den of Lions: Memoirs of Seven Years*. The actor Christopher Reeves 📖 became paralyzed from the neck down as a result of an accident and had to endure a very confining isolation. His courage and determination to continue the creative use of his many talents was inspirational. Although Nelson Mandela endured the limitations and anguish of his years in prison, he became an exceptional orator, leader, and humanitarian. Anthony Sampson has written a fascinating autho-rized autobiography of Mr. Mandela. You may wish to investigate these people's stories and develop a personal response such as writing a poem or recording their kind of experience in a creative way.

On Being an Introvert

What if you are a "loner," an introvert who simply enjoys and prefers solitude and sometimes requires an extensive amount of isolation? It may be natural for you to use reading, watching TV, and using the Internet as a replacement for the real world. However, these kinds of passive experi-ences are not real thing. When you need a clear picture of the world as it is, you have to march, wade, stride, crawl, or walk out into it.

Consider the difference in the impact of seeing pictures of a blood-ied stranger versus actually bandaging a friend who is injured and moaning. There is also a major difference between reading a joke versus telling that joke to someone who is waiting for the punch line. Knowing that rap music exists is a quite dissimilar experience than listening to it. In order to develop genuine empathy for others, you need to be where the action is—involved in face-to-face human interactions. True substi-tution for sociability is impossible.

Do you question whether most of your knowledge of humanity is based upon hearsay or second-hand information? Are you willing and able to directly judge and understand people? Or are you content to simply use an external norm as a measure of what you can and will do in response to being with people? Do you realize that how you value others will influence how they value you? Have you thought about developing a balance between solitude and social mingling in your life so that they are in reason-able proportion? These are serious questions that require serious thought. If you are an introvert, such contemplation may be an enjoyable task.

On Being an Extrovert

What if you are an extrovert? If so, then the outside world attracts you, and you are extremely sociable. This personality trait may be an inborn predisposition, or it could result from imitating the habits of family members or from limited opportunities for solitude because of crowded living conditions. However, the extent of your immersion in other people and activities can actually be a problem. You may have plenty of direct experience, but it might have little personal meaning. You tend to avoid the contemplative solitude that is needed to examine your experiences in a way that is significant to you. Asking yourself such self-examining questions as: "Why is this beautiful? Where can I use that? What should I keep?" is important because it helps in developing your persona, in your becoming someone you would want to have as a friend.

As an extrovert, you may need to ask yourself if you are afraid to be alone. If solitude frightens you, then you should ask why. You will be with you for the rest of your life. No one else could be a better friend. Your inner self is the only one fully aware of your unique and total history, capable of understanding you, able to help you laugh at yourself, often chattering in response to sensory input. This inner self really desires serious talk and meaningful conversation, at least occasionally. Why not indulge yourself sometimes, quietly and alone?

Finding a Balance

Although labels are applied as easily to both canned groceries and people, the actual content inside is more complex than indicated by a label. Probably no one could be completely introverted or extroverted. You are occasionally more one than the other, and that adds a challenge to each day and maybe even to each moment of each day. What label is most suitable for you right now?

There are two extremes in living styles that relate to solitude. One is the simple cabin-in-the-woods experience of Henry David Thoreau 📖. The other extreme is the opulent hideaway of celebrities, where the privacy of the occupants is protected by many employees. Some examples of the latter have included the homes of William Randolph Hearst 📖, Frank Sinatra 📖, Elvis Presley 📖, and Bill Gates 📖. You may realize that, despite their extreme differences, the common similarity is the real need to be alone—at least occasionally.

Dr. Jane Piirto, in her book *Understanding Creativity,* includes a section on solitude. Among other ideas, she states:

> *In creative people's lives, their work is often the most important thing. Others achieve inner peace through their spirituality, through contemplations of nature, art, or music,*

or through exercise. All of these are usually done alone. Creative people may be solitary, but that doesn't make them neurotic or unhappy.

Time alone, apart from others, may be essential for the concentration needed to write, to bring forth that which is new or invented, and to live fully. The imaginative eye can be turned inward, seeking truth internally, possibly with a desire to better see and serve society from a perspective of isolation. It may be that the most sublime reaches of creative people occur in narrowed spaces, with limited human contacts, and in a stillness great enough to make their own heartbeats noisily obvious.

Now, in solitude, record your response to the ideas of this chapter in your personal notebook.

Summary

- Solitude and socializing are both common human needs.

- The proportion of solitude in your life is important.

- Your need and opportunities for solitude vary.

- Meditation can help you develop personally and creatively.

- Self-chosen solitude can enhance your creativity.

- It is possible to make creative use of enforced solitude.

- You can use various techniques to decrease the stress of social isolation.

- You can be solitary, creative, and happy.

Words of Wisdom

Our language has wisely sensed the two sides of being alone. It has created the word "loneliness" to express the pain of being alone. And it has created the word "solitude" to express the glory of being alone.
— Paul Tillich

Talents are best nurtured in solitude; character is best formed in the stormy billows of the world.
— J. W. von Goethe

Solitude is as needful to the imagination as society is wholesome for the character.
— James Russell Lowell

When we cannot bear to be alone, it means we do not properly value the only companion we have from birth to death—ourselves.
— Eda LeShan

Friendship needs no words—it is loneliness relieved of the anguish of loneliness.
— Dag Hammarskjold

The artist, however faithful to his personal vision of reality, becomes the last champion of the individual mind and sensibility against an intrusive society and an officious state. The great artist is thus a solitary figure. He has, as (Robert) Frost said "a lover's quarrel with the world."
— John F. Kennedy

People are lonely because they build walls instead of bridges.
— J. F. Newton

To be alone is to be different. To be different is to be alone.
— Suzanne Gordon

If a man does not keep pace with his companions, perhaps it is because he hears a different drummer. Let him step to the music which he hears, however measured or far away.
– Henry David Thoreau

Loneliness is the poverty of self; solitude is the richness of self.
– May Sarton

I love people. I love my family, my children…but inside myself is a place where I live all alone and that's where you renew your springs that never dry up.
– Pearl S. Buck

Solitude is painful when one is young, but delightful when one is more mature.
– Albert Einstein

Solitude is such a potential thing. We hear voices in solitude we never hear in the hurry and turmoil of life; we receive counsels and comforts we get under no other condition.
– Amelia E. Barr

Being solitary is being alone well: being alone luxuriously immersed in doings of your own choice, aware of the fullness of your own presence rather than of the absence of others. Because solitude is an achievement.
– Alice Koller

The whole value of solitude depends upon one's self; it may be a sanctuary or a prison, a haven of repose or a place of punishment, a heaven or a hell, as we ourselves make it.
– John Lubbock

Chapter 23

All of Your Tomorrows: The Road Ahead

All of your tomorrows begin with today. What you do—or don't do—today will have an effect on your future; however, the extent of this influence may not be obvious for a long time. Considerable wisdom is required to see the cause and effect of each day's activities. You may have a strong tendency to believe that the activities of other people and circumstances are the most powerful influences on you. However, many times it is *your* attitude, actions, and effort that determine the outcome of a situation.

- Develop a "take charge" attitude; be in command of yourself and maintain a determination to reach your goals.

- Let your dreams and desires sweep away your past uncertainties.

- Work optimistically for a future that can satisfy your best inner self.

Predicting the future is a challenging and uncertain process. At present, the future seems certain to include greater use of computers and wireless technology. There is growing concern about the supply, commercial use, and distribution of natural resources. Changes appear certain in financial institutions, transportation systems, and social services. Bioengineering, geological exploration, computer system development, health sciences technology, and agricultural technology seem to have great career potential. There always is a need for people with abilities, ideas, and willingness to work hard in *any* field.

It can be tempting to make predictions, but it is sobering to realize the extent to which past predictions have failed. Two examples are especially interesting—first, the predicted near-destruction of humanity by starvation in the mid-950s, and second, the prediction of an overabundance of electrical energy by the mid-1970s. If the former had come true, the latter would certainly be true—assuming that the remnant population maintained existing power plants. Both predictions were based on what was currently sound knowledge at that time.

The starvation concept arose in the 19th century as a result of examining converging graphs of rising population and diminishing sources of fixed nitrogen needed for plant growth and food stores. It overlooked the possibility of technological invention, however, which did occur. The chemical fixation of nitrogen by the Haber 📖 process in the early 20th century permitted the manufacture of chemical fertilizers and thus averted the starvation crisis.

Excess power production was an extrapolation based on the initial stages of nuclear power plant design. It was thought that electric power would become so plentiful and cheap that metering for household use would be unnecessary. This prediction failed for many reasons, including an unrealistic assessment of total production costs.

Preparing for a Less than Certain Future

What can you do to prepare for a less-than-certain tomorrow? It can be daunting not knowing what is to come, but rest assured that there will be many novel opportunities. The following suggestions can help. You may recognize a number of them because of their inclusion in previous chapters.

- ▣ Make an effort to learn as much as possible about people, their nature, and their needs. Take a good psychology course, educate yourself by using Internet and library facilities, and become a careful observer. Study yourself—but beware of becoming too self-concerned.

- ▣ Remember that any change disturbs more than the immediate item or circumstance. Try to evaluate what has been called the "butterfly effect" 📖 or "ripple effect."

- ▣ When something goes wrong or needs changing, seek advice from at least one impartial source (it could be a person or a book) *and* from someone who knows you and cares about you. Use the advice when possible.

- Begin accumulating a personal money fund, and develop a good credit history. They will provide a cushion in the event of a needed career change or any other upset. Treat money with respect, not avarice. Be aware of the social implications of your expenditures. Your spending becomes a statement of support for a product, an event, or anything else. Somehow, somewhere, money has a human value in goods produced or work expended. Therefore, in spending money, you are using an exchange of human effort.

- Read local newspapers and, if possible, at least one national paper, such as the *New York Times* or the *Washington Post*.

- Read at least one foreign journal or newspaper on a regular basis. Explore the Internet and the many foreign publications available online. Check the public library for possibilities. Other parts of the world have different opinions about us and the world. By comparison with indigenous papers and magazines, the differences in points of view and values may be useful in assessing demographics and future political changes.

- Maintain membership in at least one group that is active in community affairs. This gives you a way to scan the horizon for changes within your immediate area.

- On a regular basis (use your personal calendar), evaluate your present circumstances as they relate to your long-range goals. Use creative thinking to figure out possible changes. Do this when you are in a good mood.

- Live each day as fully and as honorably as you can—perhaps as though each day might be your last one.

- Read—regularly, widely, and carefully.

- Evaluate the importance or value of anything by using a time perspective. Ask yourself, "How important will this be in a week, a month, a year?"

- Attend conferences and workshops. Take courses. Write. Create. Publish. Speak. Share your ideas. Explore the Internet.

- Regularly and rigorously examine your code of ethics and your current behaviors, as well as your working and living circumstances. Do they agree? If not, what should you do?

- Maintain a social life. Beware of isolation, but value solitude.

- Attend cultural events as often as possible. Remember that the art world, for example, not only mirrors the present, it often gives a glimpse of the future.

- Become active politically. Political processes shape the future. Volunteer work is an excellent way to gather insights.

- If change suddenly overwhelms you, remember to gather up your confidence. You are okay. Whatever happens, know that you *will* manage.

Allegorical Symbolism and You

One of the primary purposes of this book is to help you respond creatively to opportunities. This last exercise involves an opportunity to decode symbols in an allegory. Understanding symbolism is the first step toward interpreting this allegory.

Just knowing that symbols exist does little to enhance creative efforts. It is the invention of symbols and the subsequent investigation of meaning that is associated with creative acts. Symbolism, when used in literary contexts, involves the use of specific words and phrases to represent thoughts, ideas, or objects. Excavating meaning from writing or other symbolic usage literally converts concepts to your authorship or ownership. Your sensitivity to hidden ideas and your interest in decoding that which is mysterious can be a pleasing and useful adventure.

You may also enjoy decoding various artworks of known allegorical origin. For example, Thomas Cole's series of paintings called "The Voyage of Life" 📖 at the National Gallery of Art in Washington, D.C. symbolically represents the four stages of life. Many prints from the 18th and 19th centuries likewise carry allegorical significance. Certain plays, many poems, and some musical compositions have been created with concealed meaning. Your sensitivity to hidden ideas and your interest in decoding that which is mysterious can be a pleasing and useful adventure.

The following allegory is a symbolic narrative. Its most interesting aspect is not the story line; it is the meaning that you can assign to it. Your sense of the code will be affected by your experiences, knowledge, feelings, and beliefs. This decoding process varies from person to person, and there are no absolutely right or wrong answers. At another time, even your interpretation may change.

As a suggestion, read the entire story and set it aside for a few days. At a second reading, imagine how you could connect the words to an overall meaning or theme. Record your ideas on paper or computer. You might try writing your own allegory or perhaps finding another allegory to interpret. Many very powerful ones were written during ancient Greek and Roman times and can be found in classical literature.

The Hourglass

A piece of earth, a sand grain of quartz lifted skyward and swirled a great distance, enters the complex town of Eversame one morning. It bounces against a long fence; then it drops into a groove in a toy chest. The chest, which is painted red and blue, is lodged in a clump of wild asparagus.

The next spring, a woman searching for food mutters, "that careless child." As she rubs the toy box clean, the sand grain falls and clings to her sock. At home, in the wash water from her clothes, the sand grain sinks into the water table. There, the tiny particle spends years before being carried to a stream edge.

On one clouded fall day, the same sand grain sticks to the side of the yellow boot of an old man. While he patiently sits on the stream bank fishing, he dreams—remembering childhood friends and their games with the contents of a red and blue toy chest. Walking back to the highway, the sand grain drops from his boot. On the next windy day, the grain is conveyed by a car tire to an unknown destination.

One Possible Interpretation

One possible interpretation, using the theme of ideas, follows (phrases and terms from the allegory are italicized):

A piece of earth, a sand grain of quartz—an idea—*lifted skyward and swirled a great distance*—arrives from outside (foreign)—*enters the complex town of Eversame one morning*—the town, as suggested by its title, has a social structure not receptive to change and strange ideas. *It bounces against a long fence*—a barrier to ideas or a boundary that both includes and excludes ideas—*then it drops into a groove in a toy chest. The chest, which is painted red and blue, is lodged in a clump of wild asparagus*—reception of a new idea associated with youth (toy chest) as well as "wild" food for thought (asparagus).

The next spring, a woman searching for food mutters, "that careless child"—concern that the toy box was lost or abandoned; an act against social standards? Or perhaps it is an indication of the limits of play. *As she rubs the toy box clean, the sand grain falls and clings to her sock*—the sand grain, the idea, attaches to the covering of her feet, the part most capable of physically moving self in a new direction. *At home, in the wash water from her clothes*—inability, chosen or accidental, to keep the new concept—*the sand grain sinks into the water table*—ideas not accepted, worked with, or neglected are stored somewhere merely needing discovery. *There, the tiny particle*—initially ideas may seem small, unimportant—*spends years*—some ideas, especially those of social change, require a long time prior to acceptance, especially in places like Eversame—*before being carried to a stream edge*—an active proponent of an idea is needed to release it into a current stream of thought.

On one clouded fall day—for most people, less than ideal conditions exist for some idea transfers—*the same sand grain sticks to the side of the yellow boot*—ideas as mere "footnotes" to living—*of an old man*—now have three persons mentioned and more implied in the existence of a town. If they are archetypal, what do they represent in a place like Eversame? Woman: food supplier, child care, cleaning; Child: play, learning; Man: employed (yellow boots), food supplier, recreation. Could ideas change these roles for some people or some times? *While he patiently sits on the stream bank fishing*—anyone of any age can go fishing for ideas—*he dreams—remembering*—more active effort needed to hold onto ideas—*childhood friends and their games with the contents of a red and blue toy chest*—primary colors (including yellow boots) represent ideas held in primary esteem. *Walking back to the highway, the sand grain drops from his boot*—leaving that idea behind. *On the next windy day, the grain is conveyed by a car tire to an unknown destination*—an optimistic ending; the unrecognized idea still exists, waiting for discovery.

Could this allegory be decoded in a better way, perhaps using a dual theme of time and ideas? Write some responses to this decoding in your personal notebook. You could make your own analysis of *The Hourglass*, satisfying your viewpoints. *The Next Sunrise*, which follows, is another allegory for your interpretation.

The Next Sunrise

Imagine that you are walking in a vast meadow with the morning song of birds orchestrating pleasure. Distantly, you perceive what appears to be a huge, white rock tilted against a blue horizon. As you head toward it, the sky darkens, a tumble of rain blurs the distance, and you slog onward. There is no shelter.

When the hot sun dries you, the rock reappears—no longer white, and also smaller in size. You must have walked away from it during the storm. You long to talk to someone, but there is no one in sight.

Should you continue? Is it that important? You proceed toward the rock. A small toad hops away from you, reminding you to be careful of your steps. A tiny piece of foil catches your eye. You shape it gently and prop it on top of a daisy.

Now the rock begins to have a shape like a tablet, and its long shadow almost touches you. The sun sets, and the colors suffuse the long grass blades. An image of green daggers troubles you.

You reach the rock just in time to see faint lettering chipped in it—your name shocks you for a moment. Then you realize that everyone has the same name—Human. With a sense of satisfaction, you lean against it for a comfortable sleep.

The next sunrise glints its beam from the foil to a sleepy toad.

What is next? What will your next sunrise bring?

Summary

▣ The future is yours—dotted, striped, green, tough, rocky, tender, flat, tumultuous—all yours!

Words of Wisdom

The way I see it, if you want a rainbow, you gotta put up with the rain.
— Dolly Parton

I like living. I have sometimes been wildly, despairingly, acutely miserable, racked with sorrow, but through it all I still know quite certainly that just to be alive is a grand thing.
— Agatha Christie

I began to have an idea of my life, not as the slow shaping of achievement to fit my preconceived purposes, but as the gradual discovery and growth of a purpose which I did not know.
— Joanna Field

Talent is the gift plus the passion—a desire to succeed so intense that no force on earth can stop it.
— Neil Simon

My interest is in the future—because I'm going to spend the rest of my life there.
— Charles F. Kettering

Life, for all its agonies of despair and loss and guilt, is exciting and beautiful, amusing and artful and endearing, full of liking and love, at times a poem and a high adventure, at times noble and at times very gay; and whatever (if anything) is to come after it—we shall not have this life again.
— Rose Macaulay

Who in the world am I? Ah, that's the great puzzle.
— Lewis Carroll

The best way to make your dreams come true is to wake up.
— J. M. Power

When it comes to the future, there are three kinds of people: those who let it happen, those who make it happen, and those who wonder what happened.
— John M. Richardson

The future is called "perhaps," which is the only possible thing to call the future. And the only important thing is not to allow that to scare you.
— Tennessee Williams

Leaders establish the vision for the future and set the strategy for getting there.
— John P. Kotter

The future belongs to those who see possibilities before they become obvious.
— John Sculley

Learn from the past, look to the future, but live in the present.
— Petra Nemcova

Epilogue

For You

Oh, try – let your voice come
Lilting with full sounds for
Metal gilting any dark marks
On the pure golden larking
That must cover the dust of living.
Oh cry – with a song that
Slipping tantalizes the air
By ripping at the stillness
In words and rhythms
To remove the rust of living.
Oh sigh – a breath let loose
Aching any answer with
Love and caring that will
Augur and argue meaning
Central to the crust of living.
Oh fly – gather cirrus and skybolts
Flinging energy with focus
Enough kindling of desires
To challenge your faculties
And heart touch the thrust of living.

With love,
BJE

All-Time Great Books

Here are some books that, in my opinion, contain timeless ideas and extensive wisdom. I hope that you will find opportunities to read some or all of them.

Aeschylus: *Oresteia; Prometheus Bound*

Aristophanes: *The Frogs; Plutus; Lysistrata; The Clouds*

Aristotle: *The Poetics; Ethics; The Art of Poetry*

Augustine: *Confessions*

Aurelius: *Meditations*

The Bible: *Genesis; Amos; Job; Matthew; John; Romans*

Cervantes: *Don Quixote*

Dante: *Inferno*

Dostoyevsky: *Crime and Punishment*

Euripides: *Electra; Iphigenia in Taurus; Hippolytus; Medea; The Bacchae*

Fielding: *Tom Jones*

Goethe: *Faust, Part 1 and 2*

Herodotus: *The Persian Wars*

Homer: *Iliad; Odyssey*

Lucretius: *On the Nature of Things*

Machiavelli: *The Prince*

Milton: *Paradise Lost*

Moliere: *Tartuffe; The Misanthrope; The Physician in Spite of Himself; School for Wives*

Montaigne: *Essays*

Plato: *Ion; Apology; Republic; Phaedo; Symposium*

Rabelais: *Gargantua and Pantagruel*

Rousseau: *Confessions*

Shakespeare: *Henry IV, Parts 1 and 2; King Lear; Anthony and Cleopatra; The Tempest*

Sophocles: *Oedipus the King; Antigone; Ajax; Philoctetes*

Spinoza: *Ethics*

Swift: *Gulliver's Travels*

Thucydides: *The History of the Peloponnesian War*

Virgil: *Aeneid*

Voltaire: *Candide*

Recommended Reading

These are books that have meant a lot to me. You may find them interesting as well, and perhaps you can start a list of books that are special to you or that you want to read.

Agosin, M. (Ed.). Giachetti, M. (Translator). (1993). *A Gabriela mistral reader.* Fredonia, NY: White Pine Press.

Ayan, J. (1997). *Aha! 10 ways to free your creative spirit and find your great ideas.* New York: Crown Trade Paperbacks.

Baskin, Y. (1997). *The work of nature: How the diversity of life sustains us.* Washington, DC: Island Press.

Bernstein, P. L. (1996). *Against the gods: The remarkable story of risk.* New York: John Wiley & Sons.

Bohle, B. (1986). *The home book of American quotations.* New York: Gramercy.

Bronowski, J. (1973). *The ascent of man.* Boston/Toronto: Little, Brown & Co.

Coleman, A. M. (1999). *What is psychology?* (3rd ed.). London: Routledge.

Dana, D. (1961). I. Baltimore: Johns Hopkins University Press.

Dillard, A. (1990). *The writing life.* New York: Harper Perennial.

Doerger, F. G. (1997). *Welcome to the real working world: What every employee must know to succeed.* Santa Monica, CA: General Publishing Group.

Einstein, A. (1949). *The world as I see it.* New York: Philosophical Library.

Einstein, A. (1985). *Ideas and opinions.* New York: Crown

Eiseley, L. (1978). *The star thrower.* London: Wildwood House.

Epstein, J. (Ed.). (1997). *The Norton book of personal essays.* New York: Norton & Co.

Exley, H. (Ed.). (1993). *The best of women's quotations.* New York: Exley.

Fieve, R. R. (1997). *Moodswing* (2nd ed.). New York: Bantam.

Foster, H. W., Jr. (1997). *Make a difference.* New York: Scribner.

Frankl, V. E. (2006). *Man's search for meaning.* Uckfield, East Sussex: Beacon Press.

Fukuyama, F. (1992). *The end of history and the last man.* New York: Free Press.

Gamez, G. (1996). *Creativity: How to catch lightning in a bottle.* Los Angeles: Peak.

Garner, A. (1991). *Conversationally speaking: Tested new ways to increase your personal and social effectiveness.* Los Angeles: Lowell House Contemporary Books.

Gell-Mann, M. (1995). *The quark and the jaguar. Adventures in the simple and the complex.* New York: W. H. Freeman & Co.

Gould, S. J. (1996). *Full house: The spread of excellence from Plato to Darwin.* New York: Harmony Books.

Gould, S. J. (1997). *Questioning the millennium: A rationalist's guide to a precisely arbitrary countdown.* New York: Harmony Books.

Griffin, J. (1994). *How to say it best: Choice words, phrases, and model speeches for every occasion.* New York: Prentice Hall.

Hawking, S. W. (1988). *A brief history of time: From the big bang to black holes.* New York: Bantam.

Hawking, S. W. (1996). *The nature of space and time.* Princeton, NJ: Princeton University Press.

Haynes, M. E. (1998). *Effective meeting skills: A practical guide for more productive meetings.* Los Altos, CA: Crisp Publications.

Hirsch, E. D. (1987). *Cultural literacy: What every American needs to know.* Boston: Houghton Mifflin.

Hoff, R. (1992). *I can see you naked.* Kansas City, MO: Andrews & McMeel.

Huang, C. A., & Lynch, J. (1995). *Mentoring: The Tao of giving and receiving wisdom.* New York: HarperCollins.

Kent, P. (1996). *The complete idiot's guide to the Internet.* Indianapolis, IN: Que.

Kitwood, T. (1990). *Concern for others: A new psychology of conscience and morality.* New York: Routledge.

Kottler, J. (1990). *Private moments, secret selves.* Los Angeles: Jeremy P. Tarcher.

Luoma, J. R. (1999). *The hidden forest: The biography of an ecosystem.* New York: Henry Holt & Co.

Madigan, C. O., & Elwood, A. (1983). *Brainstorms and thunderbolts: How creative genius works.* New York: MacMillan.

May, R. (1983). *The discovery of being: Writings in existential psychology.* New York: W. W. Norton & Co.

McGrath, C. (Ed.). (1998). *A hundred years of authors, ideas and literature from the New York Times.* New York: Times.

Morse, J. D. (1979). *Old master paintings in North America.* New York: Abbeville Press.

Mueller, L., & Reynolds, J. D. (1990). *Creative writing: Forms and techniques.* Lincolnwood, IL: National Textbook.

Mullis, K. (1998). *Dancing naked in the mind field.* New York: Pantheon.

Parini, J. (1999). *Robert Frost: A life.* New York: Henry Holt & Co.

Peacock, M. (1998). *How to read a poem and start a poetry circle.* New York: Riverhead.

Plotnik, A. (1996). *The elements of expression.* New York: Henry Holt & Co.

Post, E. L. (1990). *Emily Post on invitations and letters.* New York: Harper & Row.

Post, E. L., & Coles, J. M. (1986). *Emily Post talks with teens about manners and etiquette.* New York: Harper & Row.

Random House. (1996). *Random House power vocabulary builder.* New York: Author.

Redway, K. (1997). *How to be a rapid reader: 6 steps to increased speed and concentration.* Lincolnwood, IL: National Textbook.

Rozakis, L. E. (1997). *The complete idiot's guide to creative writing.* New York: Alpha.

Sarton, M. (1973). *Journal of a solitude.* New York: Norton & Co.

Savant, M. V., & Fleischer, L. (1990). *Brain building in just 12 weeks.* New York: Bantam.

Scheibe, K. E. (2000). *The drama of everyday life.* Boston: Harvard University Press.

Seldes, G. (1985). *The great thoughts.* New York: Ballantine.

Sheehy, E. P. (Ed.). (1986). *Guide to reference books* (10th ed.). Chicago/ London: American Library Association.

Sherman, R., & Seldon, P. (1997). *The complete idiot's guide to classical music.* New York: Alpha.

Siepmann, K. B. (Ed.). (1987). *Benet's reader's encyclopedia* (3rd ed.). New York: Harper & Row.

Siever, L. J. (1997). *The new view of self: How genes and neurotransmitters shape your mind, your personality, and your health.* New York: MacMillan.

Simpson, J. B. (1988). *Simpson's contemporary quotations.* Boston: Houghton Mifflin.

Sinatra, S. T. (1997). *Optimum health: A natural lifesaving prescription for your body and mind.* New York: Bantam.

Smith, H. W. (1994). *The 10 natural laws of successful time and life management: Proven strategies for increased productivity and inner peace.* New York: Warner.

Storr, A. (1988). *Solitude: A return to the self.* New York: Ballantine.

Szymborska, W. (1998). *Poems: New and collected 1957-1997.* New York: Harcourt Brace.

Tate, J. (1991). *Selected poems.* Hanover/London: University Press of New England.

Trilling, L., & Weiseltier, L. (Eds.). (2000). *The moral obligation to be intelligent: Selected essays.* New York: Farrar, Straus & Giroux.

Tucker, T. (1995). *Brainstorm!: The stories of twenty American kid inventors.* New York: Farrar, Straus & Giroux.

Walters, L. (1993). *Secrets of a successful speaker: How you can motivate, captivate and persuade.* New York: McGraw-Hill.

Warren, R. P. (1996). *Sixty years of American poetry: Celebrating the anniversary of the Academy of American Poets.* New York: Harry N. Abrams.

Wechsler, H. J. (1967). *Great prints et printmakers.* New York: Harry N. Abrams.

References in Chapters

Anderson, T. A. (1993). *Den of lions: Memoirs of seven years*. New York: Crown.

Austin, J. (2006). *Zen-brain reflections*. Cambridge, MA: MIT Press.

Austin, L. (2001). *What's holding you back: 8 Critical choices for women's success*. New York: Basic.

Berg, H. S., & Conyers, M. (1998). *Speed reading: The easy way*. New York: Barron's.

Bolles, R. N. (2006). *What color is your parachute? 2007*. Berkley, CA: Ten Speed Press.

Breaugh, J. A. (1981). Relationships between recruiting sources and employee performance, absenteeism and work attitude. *Academy of Management Journal, 24*(1), 142-147.

Buchholz, D. (2002). *Heal your headache*. New York: Workman.

Carson, R. (1987). *Silent spring* (25th anniversary issue). Boston: Houghton Mifflin.

Champy, J., & Nohria, N. (2001). *The arc of ambition: Defining the leadership journey*. New York: Wiley.

Chopra, D. (2005). *The book of secrets: Unlocking the hidden dimensions of your life*. New York: Three Rivers Press.

Covey, S. (2003). *The 7 habits of highly effective teens*. New York: Fireside.

Covey, S. (2003). *The 7 habits of highly effective teens personal workbook*. New York: Fireside.

Covey, S. R. (2004). *The seven habits of highly effective people*. New York: Free Press.

Csikszentmihalyi, M. (1998). *Finding flow: The psychology of engagement with everyday life*. New York: Basic Books.

Duke, P., & Hochman, G. (1993). *A brilliant madness: Living with manic depression illness*. New York: Bantam.

Dyer, W. (2005). *The power of intention*. London: Hay House.

Eliot, T. S. (1955). *The Wasteland and other poems*. San Diego, CA: Harvest.

Epstein, J. (1989). *Ambition, the secret passion*. Chicago: Ivan R. Dee.

Frankl, V. E. (2006). *Man's search for meaning*. Uckfield, East Sussex: Beacon Press.

Gephart, R., & Wessel, M. (1999). *An even better place: America in the 21st century*. New York: Public Affairs.

Girard, J. (1986). *How to sell anything to anybody.* New York: Warner.

Goldman, D. R. (Ed.). (1999). *American College of Physicians complete home medical guide.* New York: DK.

Goleman, D. (2006). *Emotional intelligence: Why it can matter more than IQ* (10th ed.). New York: Bantam.

Hansen, R. S., & Hansen, K. (2007). *What do employers really want? Top skills and values employers seek from job-seekers.* Quintessentnial Careers: Your Job Starts Here. Retrieved August 14, 2007, from www.quintcareers.com/job_skills_values.html

Herriot, J. (1974). *All things bright and beautiful.* New York: St. Martin's Press.

Keller, H. A. (1903). *The story of my life.* New York: Doubleday.

Keller, H. A. (1957). *The open door.* Garden City, NY: Doubleday.

Kennedy, J. F. (1994). *Profiles in courage.* New York: HarperCollins.

Kennedy, J. F. (1994). *Profiles in courage: Young reader's memorial edition.* New York: Harper & Row.

Kohl, P. (1988). *Hole in the garden wall.* Beachwood, Ohio: Cyrano Guildmaster.

Kump, P. (1998). *Breakthrough rapid reading.* New York: Prentice Hall

Liebman, J. L. (1998). *Peace of mind: Insights on human nature that can change your life.* Yucca Valley, CA: Citadel.

Likoff, L., & Romanosky, N. (Eds.). (2007). *Encyclopedia of career and vocational guidance* (14th ed.). Chicago: Ferguson.

Lindbergh, A. M. (1991). *Gift from the sea.* New York: Random House.

McGraw, P. C. (2006). *Life strategies: Doing what works, doing what matters.* New York: Hyperion.

Molloy, J. T. (1984). *Molloy's live for success.* New York: Bantam.

Molloy, J. T. (1988). *John T. Molloy's new dress for success.* New York: Warner.

Molloy, J. T. (1996). *The new woman's dress for success.* New York: Warner.

Occupational Outlook Handbook (annual publication). Washington, DC: Superintendent of Documents, Government Printing Office.

Piirto, J. (2004). *Understanding creativity.* Scottsdale, AZ: Great Potential Press.

Pitino, R., & Reynolds, B. L. (1998). *Success is a choice: Ten steps to overachieving in business and life.* New York: Broadway.

Prentiss, C. (2006). *Zen and the art of happiness.* Malibu, CA: Power Press.

Reivich, R., & Shatté, A. (2002). *The resilience factor: 7 keys to finding your inner strength and overcoming life's hurdles.* New York: Broadway Books.

Rozakis, L. E. (1999). *The complete idiot's guide to public speaking* (2nd ed.). New York: Alpha.

Sampson, A. (1999). *Mandela: The authorized biography.* New York: Alfred A. Knopf.

Scheele, A. M. (1996). *Skills for success: A guide to the top for men and women.* New York: Ballantine.

Seligman, M. E. P. (1995). *What you can change—and what you can't: The complete guide to successful self-improvement: Learning to accept who you are.* New York: Fawcett.

Traxel, R. G. (1978). *Manager's guide to successful job hunting.* New York: McGraw Hill.

Vital Speeches of the Day (bi-monthly publication). Mt. Pleasant, SC: City News.

Warrell, M. (2007). *Find your courage!: Unleash your potential and live the life you really want.* St. Ives, NSW: Synergy.

Woods, R. L. (1967). *Modern handbook of humor for speakers, writers, business and professional men and all who enjoy sharing humor with others.* New York: McGraw Hill.

Woolf, V. (1990). *Mrs. Dalloway.* San Diego, CA: Harvest.

Index of Names

Index of Quotations

215

"Brevity is the soul of wit." William Shakespeare 72

"Bring ideas in and entertain them..." Mark Van Doren 4

"Brush them and floss them..." American Dental Association 137

"But I want first of all..." Anne Morrow Lindbergh 123

"Chance favors the prepared mind." Louis Pasteur 25

"Churchill wrote his own speeches..." James C. Humes 118

"Civility costs nothing and buys..." Lady Mary Wortley Montagu 167

"Confidence comes not from always..." Peter T. McIntyre 45

"Conversation: A vocal competition..." Ambrose Bierce 94

"Conversation means being able to..." Dwight MacDonald 93

"Coroners (they always have the final word)..." Joseph Pursch 137

"Courage is doing what you're afraid to do..." Edward V. Rickenbacker 159

"Courage is very important..." Ruth Gordon 159

"Courage without conscience..." Robert G. Ingersoll 160

"Creativity represents a miraculous..." Norman Podhoretz 30

"Decision is a risk rooted in..." Paul Tillich 58

"Decision is a sharp knife..." Jan McKeithen 58

"Depend upon it, the brave man..." Thomas Carlyle 156

"Do good to thy friend..." Benjamin Franklin 167

"Don't compromise yourself..." Janis Joplin 85

"Don't ever let economics alone..." Denis Waitley 177

"Don't fight the problem..." George C. Marshall 58

"Don't reserve your best behavior..." Lillian Eichler Watson 168

"Don't wait until everything is just right..." Victor Mark Hansen 153

"Each day, and the living of it..." May Sarton 12

"Each day comes bearing its gift..." Anne Ruth Schabacker 167

"Eat to please thyself..." Benjamin Franklin 100

"Eloquence is logic on fire." Lyman Beecher 118

"Every great decision creates ripples..." Ben Aaronovitch 59

"Every time we start thinking..." Margaret Maron 85

"Everyone has talent. What is rare..." Erica Jong 159

"Few people know how to hold a meeting..." Robert Fuoss 109

"Find a need and fill it." Ruth Stafford Peale 151

"For, in a democracy..." John F. Kennedy 157

"For me, the creative process..." William N. Lipscomb, Jr. 137

"Friendship needs no words..." Dag Hammarskjold 187

"Give me the serenity to accept..." Reinhold Neibuhr 159

About the Author

For 25 years, **Beatrice Elyé** taught chemistry and earth sciences to high school students. She received international recognition and awards for her creative and unusual teaching style.

In her final two years of teaching, Elyé was asked to develop a program for talented and gifted students. Her purpose was to provide information to capable students to encourage them to make better use of their abilities, as well as see the joyousness of doing so. Her program had a positive effect on the participants, who became known as *The Monday Box Group*. She wrote *Teen Success: Ideas to Move Your Mind* so that she could share her unique approach with others.

Lifelong avocations of Elyé include growing rare perennials from seed, the restoration of art, and collecting Chinese porcelains. Elyé's original garden design won the National Golden Trowel award from *Garden Design* magazine.